MW01490430

Handbook of Drug Therapy in Rheumatic Disease

Pharmacology and Clinical Aspects

Handbook of Drug Therapy in Rheumatic Disease

Pharmacology and Clinical Aspects

Joe G. Hardin, Jr., M.D.

Professor, Department of Medicine, and Director, Division of Rheumatology, University of South Alabama College of Medicine, Mobile

Gesina L. Longenecker, Ph.D.

Professor and Chair, Department of Biomedical Sciences, and Associate Professor, Department of Pharmacology, University of South Alabama College of Medicine, Mobile

Little, Brown and Company
Boston/Toronto/London

Printed in the United States of America

RRD-VA

Library of Congress Cataloging-in-Publication Data

Hardin, Joe G., 1937–
    Handbook of drug therapy in rheumatic disease : pharmacology and
clinical aspects / Joe G. Hardin, Jr., Gesina L. Longenecker.—1st ed.
        p.   cm.
    Includes bibliographical references and index.
    ISBN 0-316-34604-7
    1. Rheumatism—Chemotherapy—handbooks, manuals, etc.
2. Antirheumatic agents—Handbooks, manuals, etc.   I. Longenecker,
Gesina L.   II. Title.
    [DNLM: 1. Anti-Inflammatory Agents—pharmacology—
handbooks.   2. Anti-Inflammatory Agents—therapeutic use—
handbooks.   3. Rheumatic Diseases—drug therapy—handbooks.
QV 39H262h]
RC927.H37   1992
616.7′23061—dc20
DNLM/DLC
for Library of Congress   91-33732
                                                             CIP

To my parents, husband, and children

G.L.L.

To hundreds of medical students, who over the years have taught us a great deal more than we have taught them

J.G.H.
G.L.L.

Contents

Preface

In 1991, an intriguing term was introduced to the public—*smart bomb*, a missile that is able to find and selectively destroy a highly specific target. By implication, a smart bomb is more likely to actually hit its target and less likely to cause collateral damage than one that is not smart.

Few "smart bombs" are currently available to aid in the battles against the various rheumatic diseases, a fact that embarrasses those of us who must talk about these struggles in public. Excepting the antihyperuricemic agents and a few others, the drugs addressed in *Handbook of Drug Therapy in Rheumatic Disease* blanket the inflammatory response or the immune response, or sometimes both, with a nonspecific and often incompletely understood inhibition. They hit an appropriate target surprisingly often, but the collateral damage is typically substantial. Smart bombs are on the horizon, however. More specific anti-inflammatory agents are being developed, and really smart monoclonal antibodies directed against specific components of the immune response are being clinically investigated. It is hoped that the half-life of this book will be considerably shortened by the introduction of some of these agents into clinical practice in the near future.

Numerous opinions are expressed in the clinical sections. A few (pro–salicylate therapy and con–drug therapy of osteoarthritis, for example) *may* reflect primarily those of J.G.H., but we believe that most represent the consensus of American clinical rheumatologists. Throughout this book an effort has been made to clearly label both opinion and controversy as such.

We gratefully acknowledge Sharon Sanders for her secretarial and moral support and Barbara Beyers for keeping G.L.L.'s lab going throughout the production of this book, and Marsha Mayo who took expert care of a thousand details for J.G.H. and did all the really hard work.

J.G.H.
G.L.L.

Handbook of Drug Therapy in Rheumatic Disease

Pharmacology and Clinical Aspects

1

Introduction

The field of rheumatology was born in the nineteenth century spas of Europe, matured in close association with the specialty of physical medicine, but came into its own only after a landmark advance in pharmacology. The discovery of the adrenocorticosteroids and their dramatic effect on the disease rheumatoid arthritis by Dr. Philip Hench and his associates at the Mayo clinic in 1949 gave the fledgling specialty the impetus to develop into the broad discipline that it is today. Modern rheumatology involves a diverse group of disorders (Table 1-1), most of which are initially and primarily managed pharmacologically. The variety of drugs to be discussed in this book reflects the diversity of these conditions, but some themes (the nonsteroidal anti-inflammatory drugs [NSAIDs] for example) run through most of them.

The obvious reason why the NSAIDs are used so widely in rheumatology is that most of the conditions listed in Table 1-1 have a truly inflammatory basis, the inflammation most often predominating in the synovial lining of the joint. Furthermore, many, if not most, of the conditions are of uncertain etiology, which precludes the use of a more specific therapy. Even when the cause of the inflammatory reaction is known, gout for example, an NSAID may still be indicated until a more definitive therapy has had time to be effective. The "steroidal anti-inflammatory drugs" or corticosteroids also continue to be widely used for their anti-inflammatory effect, though they are used as immunosuppressive agents as well. Consequently these two groups of drugs, the NSAIDs and the corticosteroids, will receive considerable attention in this book, though it is recognized that they have applications far beyond the field of rheumatology.

Other agents, most often associated with other fields of medicine, will not be specifically addressed here. The simple analgesics, such as acetaminophen and codeine, are widely used for rheumatic symptoms, especially in patients also taking NSAIDs regularly, but only a few aspects of their use require comment in this book. The definitive therapy of the infectious arthropathies and associated conditions is usually the proper antibiotic regimen, and a detailed discussion of antibiotics and their proper selection is best left to a monograph on infectious diseases. Primary diseases of bone, especially osteoporosis and Paget's disease, are frequently managed by rheumatologists, but hormonal manipulations play such an important role in the therapy of these disorders that they will be left to a volume on the drug therapy of endocrine diseases. Finally, the emphasis here will be on drugs that are available in the United States and approved for the conditions under consideration. Experimental therapies may be mentioned but will be discussed in detail only if it appears likely that they will be available and approved in the near future.

For many of the agents discussed in this book, the mechanism(s) of action is uncertain or completely unknown. Some were intentionally designed to structurally mimic agents of known effectiveness and many others were simply discovered serendipitously. Consequently

Table 1-1. Brief classification of the rheumatic diseases

   I. Connective tissue diseases
      A. Rheumatoid arthritis
      B. Systemic lupus erythematosus
      C. Systemic sclerosis and its variants
      D. Polymyositis/dermatomyositis
      E. Sjögren's syndrome
      F. Mixed connective tissue disease
  II. Degenerative joint diseases (osteoarthritis)
      A. Primary
      B. Secondary
 III. Spondyloarthropathies
      A. Ankylosing spondylitis
      B. Reiter's syndrome
      C. Psoriatic arthritis
  IV. Arthropathies due to or associated with infection
      A. Bacterial
      B. Viral
      C. Fungal
      D. Lyme disease
      E. Post infection arthropathies
         1. Acute rheumatic fever
   V. Crystal-induced rheumatic disorders
      A. Gout
      B. Chondrocalcinosis (pseudogout)
      C. Calcific tendinitis
  VI. Syndromes associated with vasculitis
      A. Arteritis predominating
         1. Polyarteritis nodosa
         2. Wegener's granulomatosis
         3. Giant-cell arteritis
      B. Venulitis predominating
         1. Henoch-Schönlein purpura
         2. Other hypersensitivity vasculitis syndromes
 VII. Juvenile arthritis of unknown etiology
      A. Systemic onset
      B. Pauciarticular onset
      C. Polyarticular onset
VIII. Nonarticular rheumatism
      A. Bursitis
      B. Tendinitis
      C. Enthesopathy
      D. Myofascial pain
      E. Polymyalgia rheumatica
      F. Fibromyalgia (fibrositis)
  IX. Arthritis associated with other systemic diseases
      A. Endocrinopathies
      B. Hemoglobinopathies
      C. Hemophilia
      D. Sarcoidosis
      E. Amyloidosis
      F. Others

the scientific basis of therapeutics in rheumatology very often involves double-blind controlled studies, and not pharmacology. These studies are especially important relative to diseases that are known to wax and wane and even remit spontaneously, and many rheumatic diseases fall into this category. Therefore, for many of the agents discussed in this book, as much emphasis will be given to controlled clinical trials as to basic pharmacology.

With uncommon exception and considering the exclusions listed in a preceding paragraph, the agents that are used in rheumatic disease patients fall into four major categories: the NSAIDs (including salicylates), the corticosteroids, the slow-acting agents used predominantly in rheumatoid arthritis (including the immunosuppressive drugs), and the drugs used in gout and pseudogout. Most of this book will be devoted to the basic and clinical pharmacology of the important drugs in each group, but a section at the end will briefly review the overall drug therapy of the major disorders listed in Table 1-1. Some repetition may be expected to result from this format. The reader interested in the therapy of a specific disorder might wish to read the brief section concerning it at the end of the book **first** and then review the basic and clinical pharmacology of the individual drugs recommended.

An adequate understanding of the basic mechanisms of the many drugs that are covered in subsequent chapters may be facilitated by a brief introduction to some of the mediators and processes that are their targets. The descriptions that follow are by no means complete: Additional details are provided within specific chapters and can also be found in the sources under Bibliography.

In early inflammation, neutrophils (polymorphonuclear leukocytes) and neutrophil products are prominent. Numerous conditions may result in attraction of neutrophils to a site, including cell damage, bacterial invasion, and urate crystals; the actual attraction is accomplished via elicited biochemical signals, e.g., coagulation or complement activation products, bacterial peptides, and products of the neutrophils themselves and also of other leukocytes. Activated neutrophils release leukotriene B_4 (LTB_4), prostaglandin E_2 (PGE_2), superoxide ($O_2^{\cdot}$), and proteases. Both LTB_4 and PGE_2 contribute to increased vascular permeability. Also, LTB_4 promotes additional neutrophil (and other leukocyte) participation, whereas PGE_2 and proteases are involved in cartilage and bone destruction.

In later stages of inflammation, monocytes/macrophages (M/M) become more prominent. Activation stimuli are similar to those for neutrophils. Like activated neutrophils, activated M/M can release LTB_4 and PGE_2. In addition, M/M release interleukin-1 (IL-1), an important, multifunctional mediator. In addition to direct proinflammatory actions (increased vascular permeability, angiogenesis, elicitation of PGE_2 and protease release by other cells, chemotaxis of neutrophils, stimulation of fibroblast proliferation), IL-1, together with "processed" antigen, induces a population of lymphocytes (helper lymphocytes; T-helpers) to produce interleukin-2 (IL-2). IL-2 is a mitogen that elicits proliferation of specific populations of lymphocytes, including T-lymphocytes involved in cell-mediated immunity and B-lymphocytes involved in humoral immunity. The overall stimulatory effects of IL-1, IL-2, and helper lymphocytes are

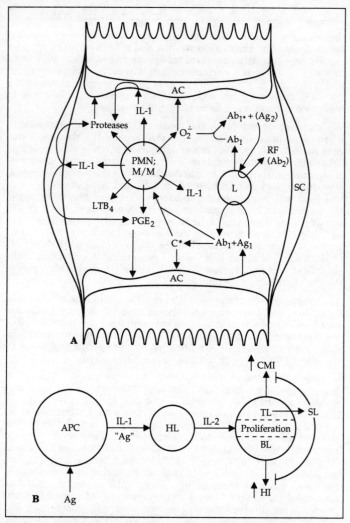

Fig. 1-1.A. Schematic of an inflamed joint showing major leukocyte (PMN, neutrophils; M/M, monocytes/macrophages; L, lymphocytes) and mediator participants. (Ab, antibody [Ab_1, primary; Ab_{1*}, modified primary; Ab_2, secondary]; AC, articular cartilage; Ag, antigen [Ag_1, primary; Ag_2, secondary (Ab_{1*})]; C, complement [*, activated cascade]; IL, interleukin [-1, -2]; LT, leukotriene [B_4]; $O_2^{\cdot-}$, superoxide anion; PG, prostaglandin [E_2]; RF, rheumatoid factor[s] [anti-IgG (IgA)]; SC, synovial cells. B. Simplified schematic showing sequence from antigen uptake to proliferation and increased effect of various lymphocytes populations. Following uptake, Ag is processed ("Ag") and presented by antigen presenting cells (APC), usually macrophages, together with released IL-1, resulting in stimulation of T-helper lymphocytes (HL) and release of IL-2. Subsets of lymphoctyes (B-, T-) proliferate, with resultant enhanced immune function (HI, humoral immunity; CMI, cell-mediated immunity). T-suppressor lymphocytes (SL) can modulate the degree of overall effect.

4

modulated by effects of another subclass of lymphocytes, i.e., suppressor lymphocytes (T-suppressors).

Involvement of antibodies in inflammation is of particular interest in that rheumatic diseases are often classified as **autoimmune**, i.e., resulting, at least in part, from inappropriate production of antibodies against "self"-antigens. Self-antibodies may result from release of (fragments of) self-macromolecules or even from accidental coincidence between foreign (e.g., bacterial) or modified self-molecules (e.g., by virus) and native self-molecules. Inappropriate production has also been proposed to result from inadequate suppressor lymphocyte function. A sustaining cycle of inflammation may be established through formation and effects of leukocyte-stimulatory immune (antigen-antibody) complexes. Modification of primary antibodies, by superoxide, for example, may elicit formation of secondary antibodies directed against the first, i.e., in formation of rheumatoid factors (anti-immunoglobulin G, A).

Interference with IL-1 can decrease its direct and lymphocyte-dependent contributions to inflammation. Interference with IL-2 can also reduce inflammation by decreasing populations of participating lymphocytes. Both mechanisms are features of some of the drugs to be discussed within this text. Other mechanisms include inhibition of the formation of PGE_2 and other related prostaglandins; inhibition of leukocyte mobility or leukocyte activation, or both; and even enhancement of lymphocyte (suppressor) function. For reference, simplified partial schematics of an inflammation cycle within a joint space and of some lymphocyte-directed actions of IL-1 are shown in Fig. 1-1.

Bibliography

Arend, W. P., and Dayer, J. M. Cytokines and cytokine inhibitors or antagonists in rheumatoid arthritis. *Arthritis Rheum.* 33:305–315, 1990.

Brain, S. D., and Williams, T. J. Leukotrienes and inflammation. *Pharmacol. Ther.* 46:57–66, 1990.

Harris, E. D. Pathogenesis of rheumatoid arthritis. *Am. J. Med.* 80(suppl. 4B):4–10, 1986.

Pettipher, E. R. Pathogenesis and treatment of chronic arthritis. *Sci. Prog.* 73:521–534, 1989.

Roberts, N. A. Free radicals, immunoglobulins and complement as mediators of inflammation. Baillieres *Clin. Rheumatol.* 2:211–232, 1988.

Uetrecht, J. Mechanism of hypersensitivity reactions: proposed involvement of reactive metabolites generated by activated leukocytes. *TIPS* 10:463–467, 1989.

Wilkinson, P. C. Cellular accumulation and inflammation. In M. M. Dale and J. C. Foreman (eds.), *Textbook of Immunopharmacology* (2nd ed). Oxford: Blackwell, pp. 209–222, 1989.

Willoughby D. A. (ed.). *Inflammation—Mediators and Mechanisms.* New York: Churchill-Livingstone, *Br. Med. Bull.* 43(2) 1987.

2

Nonsteroidal Anti-inflammatory Drugs

This chapter focuses on aspirin, the nonacetylated salicylates, and all of the nonsalicylate nonsteroidal anti-inflammatory drugs (NSAIDs) available in the United States. Acetaminophen is mentioned only briefly in the basic pharmacology section and will not be discussed clinically since it has no significant anti-inflammatory effect. The major emphases will be on the anti-inflammatory action, as opposed to the antipyretic and analgesic effects, of these agents.

Basic Pharmacology

Although several chemical classes are represented within the pharmacologic group known collectively as the NSAIDs, a common main mechanism of anti-inflammatory action can be described. This mechanism is interference with the conversion of arachidonic acid to its various biologically active, i.e., inflammation-promoting, end products. The identification of this mechanism is relatively young historically; a landmark paper from Sir John Vane's laboratory in 1971 was the official beginning.

The first identified arachidonic metabolites, described in the late 1930s, were termed **prostaglandins**, in deference to their isolation from prostatic (seminal) fluid. In recent years, the number and the chemical grouping diversity of metabolites have increased dramatically; the inclusive term **eicosanoids**, to indicate their derivation from eicosatetraenoic (arachidonic) acid, has been adopted for the various metabolites. In the following section, the metabolism of arachidonic acid is reviewed, with focus on production of two specific subgroups of metabolites, i.e., the prostanoids, which includes the prostaglandins, and also the leukotrienes and their intermediates. The site, mechanism, and consequences of NSAID action are then covered. Recent suggestions for alternate/additional mechanisms of anti-inflammatory effect are also discussed.

METABOLISM OF ARACHIDONIC ACID

It is important to recognize that arachidonic acid metabolites can be generated from most if not all types of cells, including platelets, leukocytes, vascular endothelium, synovial cells, and more. Erythrocytes, the rare exception, lack ability to convert arachidonic acid itself, although they possess an enzyme(s) for conversion of certain intermediate arachidonate metabolites, as well as end product degradative enzymes. A necessary first step in the formation of metabolites is liberation of arachidonic acid from cellular stores.

Liberation of Arachidonic Acid

Arachidonic acid (Fig. 2-1) is a 20-carbon fatty acid containing four unsaturations. It belongs to the omega-6 family of fatty acids, i.e.,

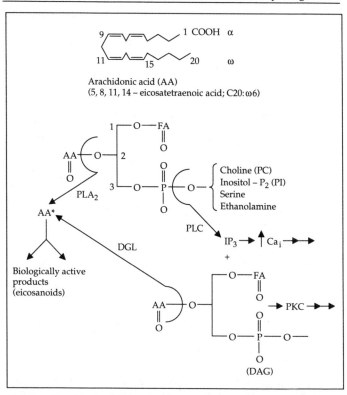

Arachidonic acid (AA)
(5, 8, 11, 14 – eicosatetraenoic acid; C20: ω6)

Fig. 2-1. Structure and liberation pathways for arachidonic acid (AA; structure at top) from membrane phospholipids. Arachidonic acid is esterified to glycerol at position 2 of the backbone of several cell membrane phospholipids, including phosphatidylcholine (PC; choline at position 3) and phosphatidylinositol (PI; inositol at position 3). Liberation of arachidonic acid by phospholiphase A_2 (PLA_2) and possibly by the sequence of phospholipase C (PLC) - diglyceride lipase, coupled to stimulus occupation of receptors initiates rapid conversation of arachidonic acid to eicosanoids, major mediators of inflammation. Intracellular signals generated by PLC action on PI amplify activity of PLA_2. (DAG, diacylglycerol; FA, fatty acid; IP_3, inositol triphosphate; ˙, availability is rate-limiting.)

a group of fatty acids in which the first double bond is encountered six positions from the omega, or noncarboxylic acid, end. The official shorthand for arachidonic acid is C:20Ω6 (or C:20n6). Arachidonic acid is found in several cell membrane phospholipid classes but is particularly abundant in phosphatidylcholine (lecithin; Fig. 2-1). Arachidonic acid is **not** abundant in free form. Indeed, availability of free arachidonic acid is the rate-limiting factor for its conversion to other products.

Liberation of arachidonic acid results from action of the stimulus(i) on specific receptors coupled to phospholipases (PL): these phospholipases, once activated, directly cleave arachidonic acid from the parent phospholipid (PLA_2), or create a diacylglycerol that is a substrate for a subsequent lipase that liberates arachidonic acid (PLC-diglyceride lipase) (Fig. 2-1). Of these two lipases, PLA_2, a membrane-associated enzyme, is generally held to be the one that is responsible for the bulk of arachidonic acid liberation. The preferred substrate for PLA_2 is phosphatidyl choline, and its site of action is the 2-position at which arachidonic acid is esterified. The activity of PLA_2 is calcium sensitive: Subsequent to interaction of stimulus with its receptors, increases in intracellular free calcium may be effected by influx of extracellular calcium through receptor-operated channels or by mobilization of calcium from intracellular storage sites, which is also a receptor-coupled event, or by a combination of these. The activity of PLA_2 may also be influenced by levels/phosphorylation state of an associated inhibitory protein as well as by levels of an (inducible) activating protein (phospholipase-activating protein; PLAP). Additional details of the regulation of PLA_2 are contained in chapter 3.

Activation of PLC is coupled to receptor occupation by stimulus(i). Although PLC activity may result in liberation of small amounts of arachidonic acid, its activity is more directly involved in signal transduction, i.e., translation of the interaction of a stimulus with its receptor into biochemical events within the cell. The preferred substrate for PLC is phosphatidyl inositol, with action at the 3-position at which inositol is esterified to the glycerol backbone through phosphates. Liberation of inositol trisphosphate, a calcium ionophore that serves to increase intracellular calcium levels through mobilization, also generates a diacylglycerol, itself an intracellular messenger that activates protein kinase C/phosphorylation reactions. The diacylglycerol may also be hydrolyzed at the 2-position by a second (diglyceride) lipase to generate arachidonic acid. The changes in intracellular calcium, and phosphorylation status of certain intracellular proteins, initiated by activation of PLC promote activation of PLA_2 and increase bulk liberation of arachidonic acid, as well as trigger other intracellular events.

The specific signals that result in liberation may differ among cell types, as a function of the receptors present. For platelets, the list of stimuli includes, but is not limited to, thrombin, complement (3a), platelet-activating factor (PAF), epinephrine, vasopressin, collagen, and adenosine diphosphate. Similar and additional stimuli (e.g., bradykinin, angiotensin [II], interleukins [IL], tumor necrosis factor [TNF_α]) can elicit liberation in vascular endothelium. For leukocytes, as a group, a partial listing of stimuli includes complement (e.g., 5a), IL, bacterial peptides (f-met-leu-phe [FMLP]), contact with bacteria/other foreign materials, PAF, and more.

Once available, arachidonic acid is rapidly converted via two major pathways, one initiated by a dioxygenase enzyme known as cyclooxygenase, the other by one or more position-specific monooxygenases known as lipoxygenase(s), and possibly via others, e.g., P450 monooxygenases. The cyclooxygenase pathway results in formation of the stable prostaglandins (e.g., $PGF_{2\alpha}$, PGE_2) and their unstable relatives (prostacyclin [PGI_2], thromboxane [TxA_2]). The lipoxygenase pathway can lead to formation of leukotrienes as well as hydroperoxy- and hydroxy- derivatives of arachidonic acid. Cyclooxygenase and lipoxygenase may compete for substrate: In in vitro systems, early production of cyclooxygenase-initiated end products has been observed, with later, more prolonged production of lipoxygenase-initiated end products.

Cyclooxygenase Pathway

Cyclooxygenase is a heme-containing enzyme that is membrane-associated, placing it in close proximity to the site of arachidonate release from membrane phospholipids. The purified enzyme has an approximate molecular weight of 66,000; its complementary DNA (cDNA) has recently been isolated. Cyclooxygenase activity has an associated (inseparable) peroxidase activity. The complex of both activities is known as prostaglandin endoperoxide synthase (PGES). As shown in the overall scheme in Fig. 2-2, two molecules of oxygen, at positions 11 and 15, are added to arachidonic acid by cyclooxygenase; these additions are accompanied by several internal structural rearrangements. The compound resulting from cyclooxygenase action, with a five-membered ring and unstable dioxygen bridge, is PGG_2. It should be noted that two of four unsaturations in arachidonic acid are eliminated as a result of cyclooxygenase action. Thus, metabolites of arachidonic acid formed via this pathway have two remaining unsaturations, a fact that is indicated in the numeric subscript of their names and abbreviations (e.g., PGE_2). The name also contains an alphabetic designation, roughly indicating purification/isolation characteristics of initially discovered ones (e.g., E = ether-extractable) or historical discovery sequence for later ones. For reference, it should be noted that biologically active metabolites can be formed from other, less abundant fatty acids, e.g., eicosatrienoic (dihomogammalinolenic) acid. These will also have two less unsaturations than the parent molecule. For dihomogammalinolenic acid, for example, one prostanoid product could be PGE_1, analogs of which are used to combat NSAID ulcerogenic actions. The actions of PGE_1 and prostacyclin are similar.

The peroxidase activity of PGES reduces the position 15 hydroperoxy group introduced by cyclooxygenase to result in a **common** intermediate, PGH_2, for formation of **all** subsequent compounds in this pathway. The action of peroxidase on its substrate results in release of an oxidant species, the identity of which is controversial. The oxidant species generated by the peroxidase activity performs the function of maintaining the "peroxide tone" required to prime the cyclooxygenase; thorough scavenging of the oxidant can result in inhibition of cyclooxygenase (Fig. 2-3). The same oxidant species may contribute to autocatalytic destruction of cyclooxygenase, and to destruction of other enzymes, e.g., prostacyclin synthase. Moderate scavenging of the oxidant can in fact prolong/enhance cyclooxygenase activity. Cooxidation reactions coupled to peroxidase are well known and have even been taken advantage of as a means of monitoring enzyme activity. It has been suggested that NADPH (the reduced form of nicotinamide-adenine dinucleotide phosphate [NADP]) can be cooxidized to NADP via coupling to PGES (Fig. 2-3), with generation of superoxide anion. Thus, metabolism of arachidonic acid initiated by cyclooxygenase could result in formation

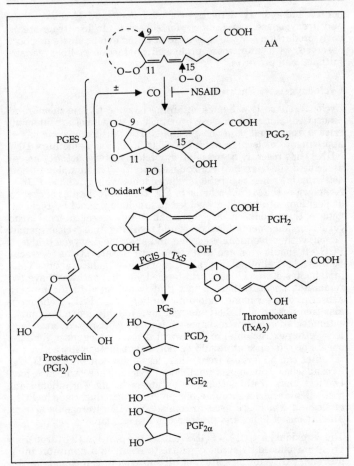

Fig. 2-2. Conversions of arachidonic acid (AA) initiated by the cyclooxygenase (CO) - peroxidase (PO) enzyme pathway. The combined CO-PO activities make up prostaglandin endoperoxide synthase (PGES). The first intermediate is PGG$_2$; the second intermediate is PGH$_2$, a common intermediate for all subsequent conversions. (—, inhibits; PG$_S$, stable prostaglandins; PGIS, prostacyclin synthase; TxS, thromboxane synthase.)

of at least two types of inflammatory mediators, prostanoids and oxidant/superoxide.

The common intermediate, PGH$_2$, can be converted to a number of end products. Conversion to the stable prostaglandins can be enzymatic or nonenzymatic. Serum albumin can nonenzymatically promote the conversion of released or leaked PGH$_2$ to PGD$_2$. Conversion of PGH$_2$ to PGE$_2$ or PGD$_2$ may proceed via an isomerase(s), sometimes referred to as **prostaglandin endoperoxide isomer-**

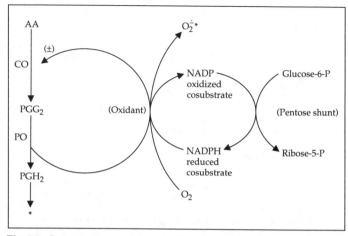

Fig. 2-3. Suggested scheme for coupling of cooxidation reactions to prostaglandin endoperoxide synthase (PGES) activity, including coupling of NADPH oxidation and generation of superoxide ($O_2^{\cdot-}$). Since the "oxidant" generated by peroxidase (PO) maintains the peroxide tone required for cyclooxygenase (CO) but is also involved in its autocatalytic destruction, coupling to cooxidations (including some to NSAIDs) has potential to stimulate (low concentrations) or inhibit (higher concentrations) PGES activity. (*, inflammation mediators.)

whereas conversion to $PGF_{2\alpha}$ may proceed via a reductase. Conversions of PGH_2 to the unstable products, prostacyclin and thromboxane, are enzymatic, catalyzed by respective synthases.

Cell types differ in the quantity as well as the end products of arachidonic acid that are produced. The spectrum of cyclooxygenase pathway end products produced by a tissue is determined by the presence and relative abundance of the enzymes that further convert PGH_2 and is somewhat characteristic for the tissue. Platelets, for example, produce mostly thromboxane, some stable prostaglandins, but no prostacyclin, whereas vascular endothelium produces prostacyclin, some stable prostaglandins, but little thromboxane. Leukocytes as a group produce relatively large amounts of PGE_2 and also some thromboxane and prostacyclin. Synovial cells release mainly PGE_2 (significant quantities).

The effects of the end products of cyclooxygenase-initiated metabolism of arachidonic acid are varied and, briefly, include, but are not limited to, the following. Some are vasoconstrictors (thromboxane, PGH_2); others are vasodilators (prostacyclin, PGE_2). Most prostanoids have weak direct ability to increase vascular permeability, but the vasodilator prostanoids additionally can enhance the permeability effects of other agents (bradykinin, histamine, other). The enhancement has been proposed to result from precapillary arteriolar dilatation. Prostacyclin and thromboxane influence the reactivity of blood platelets (inhibit and elicit aggregation, respectively). Most stimulate gastrointestinal motility, promote diarrhea, and suppress gastric acid production, but there are differing effects on cytologic stability: Prostacyclin and PGE_2 are cytoprotective and thus antiulcerogenic, whereas thromboxane reportedly is ulcerogenic and possibly cytolytic. Pain initiated by other mediators (e.g., bradykinin) is potentiated by the prostanoids. Cartilage and bone destruction are promoted by PGE_2 in particular, and PGE_2 and IL-1 may act synergistically in this regard (see also chapter 3). The latter observations have suggested that limitation of PGE_2 production may spare cartilage and bone in joint inflammatory conditions, i.e., drugs that limit PGE_2 might be classified as disease-modifying agents. Evidence supporting the suggestion in humans in vivo is currently insufficient or controversial, however.

Lipoxygenase Pathways

The lipoxygenases are cytosolic enzymes, although a loose association with, or translocation to, membrane structures has been suggested. These enzymes require activation, by increases in calcium, for example, although for at least one, an (inducible) activating protein (five lipoxygenase-activating protein [FLAP]) may also contribute.

The lipoxygenases are named by the specific site of addition of oxygen to arachidonic acid and include 5-, 8-, 9-, 11-, 12-, and 15-lipoxygenases. Individual cell types or tissues typically have only one, or sometimes two, of the lipoxygenases. Platelets and endothelium, for example, have mainly 12-lipoxygenase activity, whereas polymorphonuclear leukocytes (PMNs) have predominantly 5-lipoxygenase. Other leukocytes, e.g., monocytes, have 15-, and some 5-, lipoxygenases. Thus, the spectrum of lipoxygenase end products of a tissue partly depends on the specific lipoxygenase(s) present. The spectrum also depends on the type(s) of metabolizing enzymes for the product of the lipoxygenase activity.

The lipoxygenase that leads to the most active leukotriene end products introduces oxygen at position 5 (5-lipoxygenase); the products of 15-lipoxygenase are less active, and generation of leukotrienes from intermediates of other lipoxygenases is not well documented. The activity of 5-lipoxygenase may be modulated (increased) by levels of inflammatory mediators such as the cytokines (see chapter 3). The introduction of a single molecule of oxygen by lipoxygenase results in formation of an unstable hydroperoxy derivative (hydroperoxyeicosatetraenoic acid [HPETE]), as shown in the overall scheme in Fig. 2-4. In contrast to cyclooxygenase-initiated addition of oxygen and subsequent molecular rearrangements, introduction of oxygen by lipoxygenases does not result in any change in the number of unsaturations in the parent molecule. End products from arachidonic acid in this pathway thus have a subscript of 4, in addition to an alphabetic designation.

Also in contrast to cyclooxygenase, the lipoxygenases do not have a physically associated peroxidase activity; other cellular peroxidases, e.g., glutathione peroxidase and possibly the peroxidase of PGES, can facilitate the reduction of the hydroperoxy group, resulting in formation of the corresponding hydroxy compound (hydroxyeicosatetraenoic acid [HETE]). Lipoxygenases may have a requirement for a priming "peroxide tone" and are sensitive to antioxidant inhibition. In addition, autocatalytic destruction has been noted.

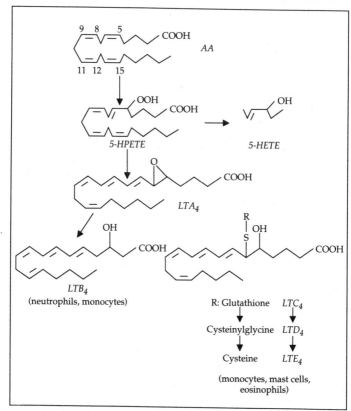

Fig. 2-4. The 5-lipoxygenase pathway for generation of leukotrienes (LT). Numbered positions on arachidonic acid (AA) indicate sites of action of other lipoxygenases. (HPETE, hydroperoxyeicosatetraenoic acid; HETE, hydroxyeicosatetraenoic acid.)

The HPETEs and HETEs are biologically active and have a range of effects, including PMN chemotaxis and promotion of adhesion. Further conversion results in formation of additional compounds with biologic activity, however. The initial product of 5-lipoxygenase, 5-HPETE, can be converted to a **common leukotriene intermediate**, i.e., LTA$_4$, by a specific synthase. This synthase may in fact be a part of 5-lipoxygenase, as it copurifies with it. The synthase converts 5-HPETE generated by the 5-lipoxygenase at a rate greater than that for exogenously added 5-HPETE, further supporting the close association between the two enzyme activities. Importantly, the activity of the synthase is rate-limiting; for any given level of 5-HPETE production, there is greater accumulation of 5-HETE than of leukotriene product.

Further conversion of LTA can occur, to LTB$_4$ in neutrophils and monocytes, for example, or to LTC$_4$, D$_4$, and E$_4$, in other cells. The latter series of compounds are collectively known as **slow-reacting substance of anaphylaxis** (SRS-A). The components of SRS-A are interconvertible, i.e., the reactions are reversible. The most prominent effects of SRS-A components include bronchoconstriction and vascular constriction, and possibly increased vascular permeability. The effects of LTB_4 include PMN degranulation and aggregation, chemokinesis and chemotaxis, and increased vascular permeability.

For completeness, it should be noted that other conversions of HPETEs are possible. For example, 12-HPETE, which is formed by platelets and vascular endothelium, can undergo conversion to compounds known as **hepoxilins**. Both 5-HPETE and 15-HPETE can be converted to lipoxins (B_3, A_3, respectively) by further action of 5-lipoxygenase-LTA synthase. A cross-product of PMNs and monocytes, i.e., 5,15-diHPETE, can also be converted to lipoxins. The contribution of these products to the overall biologic consequences of arachidonic acid metabolism is only beginning to be thoroughly investigated. One suggested action of lipoxin A is activation of protein kinase C, an action also accomplished by diacylglycerol (see Liberation of Arachidonic Acid).

DEFINITION OF NSAID CLASSES (CHEMISTRY)

Several excellent historical and comparative reviews of NSAIDs have recently been published (see Bibliography); a brief review is provided here. An excellent historical summary, as well as a survey of NSAID structures, is provided in Fig. 2-5. The usual schemes for grouping the various NSAIDs place them according to common chemical features. Using one such structural scheme, the main groups (two or more members) are the **salicylates** (including diflunisal), **pyrazolones** (phenylbutazone, oxyphenbutazone, sulfinpyrazone), **indole (indene) acetic acids** (indomethacin, sulindac, possibly tolmetin and etodolac), **phenylpropionic acids** (naproxen, ibuprofen, and others ending in -profen [-fen]), and **fenamates** and relatives (mefenamic acid, meclofenamate; diclofenac). Although there are several **oxicams**, only one is currently in use (piroxicam). An alternative structural grouping scheme consists of three main groups, each with two or more subgroups: **arylcarboxylic acids** (salicylic acids, including diflunisal; anthranilic acids, i.e., the fenamates), **arylalkanoic acids** (arylacetic acids, e.g., diclofenac; arylpropionic acids, see phenylpropionic acids; indole/indene acetic acids, i.e., indomethacin, sulindac; heteroarylacetic acids, e.g., tolmetin and etodolac), and **enolic acids** (e.g., pyrazolidinediones, phenylbutazone; oxicams).

It should be recognized that, despite the existence of distinct chemical groupings, currently available NSAIDs have in common that they are weak organic acids that are mostly ionized at physiologic pH. The more water-soluble sodium (or other) salts of several are used in preference to the free acids, when the acids are sparingly soluble or insoluble. Newer agents in development are nonacidic, and these may form a second large class when available. Most properties of NSAIDs, regardless of group or individual compound, are similar, including basic mechanism of action. Therefore, the mechanistic properties of the class are described first, followed by other general properties and descriptions by group.

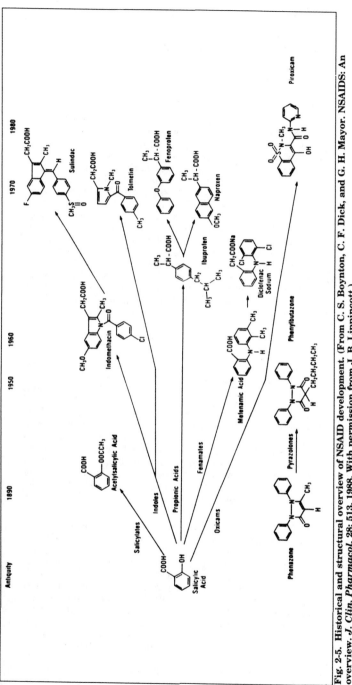

Fig. 2-5. Historical and structural overview of NSAID development. (From C. S. Boynton, C. F. Dick, and G. H. Mayor. NSAIDS: An overview. *J. Clin. Pharmacol.* 28: 513, 1988. With permission from J. B. Lippincott.)

15

SITE AND MECHANISM OF ACTION
OF NSAID ANTI-INFLAMMATORY EFFECTS

In general, NSAIDs inhibit the cyclooxygenase of the PGES complex and are without major effect at other sites, including PLA_2, lipoxygenase(s), isomerase(s), or synthases. Some possible exceptions are noted below.

The majority of NSAIDs appear to interact reversibly at a site near the active site of the enzyme (supplementary site) and some may also interact with the active site itself. This reversible interaction accounts for the observed parallelism between blood levels and effect. The most notable exception to reversibility occurs for aspirin, which, subsequent to its initial interaction with the enzyme, acetylates (a serine near the C-terminus) and permanently inactivates the enzyme. Aspirin inactivation may be limited by simultaneous presence of other NSAIDs, but this is likely due to simple competition for the binding site, rather than a specific prevention of acetylation. For most cells, replacement of inactivated cyclooxygenase molecules after a single exposure to aspirin can occur within hours and may be complete in less than a day; however, for platelets, which lack significant protein synthetic capability, the inactivation is permanent, lasting the lifespan of the cell. Full recovery of platelet function after a single usual dose (650 mg) of aspirin requires 7–10 days, the time necessary for replacement of most circulating platelets.

Although not a common strategy, attempts have been made to effect PGES inhibition by reduction of peroxide tone generated by peroxidase action. Antioxidant compounds such as MK447 and nordihydroguaiaretic acid, which are used only in vitro, probably act in this way. Several of the NSAIDs are cooxidized by PGES, including sulindac, oxyphenbutazone, and others, but it is unclear how much, if any, contribution to cyclooxygenase inhibition is made by their scavenging activity. It is worthwhile to note that acetaminophen, a phenolic derivative that is also an effective scavenger, produces platelet inhibition in a small percentage of individuals, suggesting effective inhibition of cyclooxygenase. Acetaminophen can inhibit cyclooxygenase in vitro in some tissues, but usually at high drug levels. Acetaminophen, although an effective analgesic and antipyretic compound, is essentially devoid of useful anti-inflammatory activity.

High levels of NSAIDs, such as might be used for anti-inflammatory effect, but not as used for analgesic or antipyretic effects, may have other effects in addition to cyclooxygenase inhibition. Phenylbutazone, for example, has been suggested to inhibit isomerase activity. The clinical consequence of this is unclear since phenylbutazone is a very effective inhibitor of cyclooxygenase, and, as a function of dose, there would be little PGH_2 available for conversion by isomerase. Differential effects of NSAIDs on production of individual prostanoids have been noted, however, and a contribution of effect on isomerase(s) cannot be ruled out. Some data support inhibition of PLA_2 by NSAIDs, particularly indomethacin. High levels of NSAIDs may also have some inhibitory effect on lipoxygenases. Perhaps the most intriguing possibility for high NSAID effects concerns a direct inhibition of neutrophil activation, i.e., an effect that is not dependent on inhibition of eicosanoid production.

Several general observations support anti-inflammatory effects through direct inhibitory effects on neutrophils. The first is that nonacetylated salicylates are anti-inflammatory despite the fact that they are only weak inhibitors of cyclooxygenase. Also, NSAIDs inhibit neutrophil aggregation and adhesion, and limit, to variable degrees, release of proteases and superoxide in response to chemoattractants. The inhibitory effect of NSAIDs on these processes is **not** reversed by inclusion/addition of exogenous PGE_2, rather the inhibition is **increased**; an inhibitory effect of PGE_2 on many types of leukocytes is well known. In addition, NSAIDs appear to inhibit binding of chemoattractant stimuli to specific membrane surface receptors. Last, NSAIDs may interfere with signal transduction, possibly by interacting with a G (guanine nucleotide binding) protein coupled to receptors or by changes in membrane viscosity, or both. It should be noted again that these effects of NSAIDs on neutrophils occur at concentrations greater than those required to inhibit cyclooxygenase, thus representing an **additional** mode of anti-inflammatory effect for most NSAIDs. At the same time, these neutrophil effects provide some explanation for the unanticipated anti-inflammatory effects of weak cyclooxygenase inhibitors such as the salicylates. Acetaminophen has no effect on neutrophil functions.

Immunomodulatory effects of NSAIDs on leukocytes, related to removal of leukocyte inhibitory PGE_2, have also been suggested. This is an evolving area of research. The basic premise is that NSAID-decreased PGE_2 allows for greater suppressor T function, which in turn leads to decreased production of autoantibodies. PGE_2 inhibitory effects on suppressor T cell function in vitro exceed its inhibitory effects on other immune cell populations and this presumably applies to the in vivo situation. In fact, NSAID usage in vivo in humans **has** been found to decrease serum levels of rheumatoid factor.

SPECIAL FEATURES AND MECHANISMS OF SIDE EFFECTS

Inhibition of cyclooxygenase represents an early, and common, step in the formation of **all** end products of arachidonic acid via this pathway. The effect is thus somewhat nonspecific in that some products that may not be major participants in the unwanted inflammatory process may be unnecessarily interfered with; however, the correlation between concentrations to produce inhibition of cyclooxygenase and to limit experimental inflammation is reasonably good (Table 2-1), indicating the general strategy to be rational. The ideal pharmacologic approach would necessitate explicit definition of mediators, and development of highly specific inhibitors of formative enzymes or receptor level antagonists, or both, neither of which is currently feasible. Past cyclooxygenase, effective inhibitors have been developed for thromboxane synthase and highly specific receptor level antagonists for thromboxane receptors. The latter have proven effective in limiting thromboxane effects, whereas the former may or may not be effective due to ability of PGH_2 to act as an agonist at thromboxane receptors. The thromboxane inhibitory drugs have potential utility in cardiovascular diseases, but no anti-inflammatory properties or uses have been suggested. It is also possible to pharmacologically limit prostacyclin synthase, using drugs approved for other purposes; however, the value of selectively eliminating its beneficial effects is questionable, especially including

Table 2-1. Comparison of prostaglandin synthetase inhibitory activity and anti-inflammatory potency of selected non-narcotic analgesics

Drug	Inhibition (ID_{50}) of prostaglandin synthetase (μg/mL)	Reduction (ED_{50}) of carrageenan-induced rat paw edema (mg/kg)
Indomethacin	0.06	6.5
Piroxicam	0.06	4.0
Mefenamic acid	0.17	55.0
Phenylbutazone	2.23	100.0
Acetylsalicylic acid	6.62	150.0
Acetaminophen	100	inactive

Source: H. Kalant and W. Roschlau (eds.). *Principles of Modern Pharmacology* (5th ed.). Philadelphia: Decker, 1989. P. 325. With permission from The Book Committee, Department of Pharmacology, University of Toronto.

the potential for additional effects of the inhibitory drug itself. Effective, selective, and potentially useful inhibitors of isomerase(s), and thus the stable prostaglandins, are not available but receptor level antagonists are in development.

Many (unwanted and wanted) effects of NSAIDs at sites other than the target site result from inhibition of cyclooxygenase at those sites. For cardiovascular diseases, regulation of dose may allow differential inhibition in some tissues by virtue of differences in sensitivity. For example, low-dose aspirin may effectively limit thromboxane production, and aggregation, in platelets, while leaving vascular production of prostacyclin virtually untouched. In general, the doses required for effective anti-inflammatory action exceed those to produce limitation of production of gastric protective prostanoids, platelet thromboxane, and vascular prostacyclin and PGE_2. Thus, the common "side effects" of NSAIDs, namely gastric irritation/ulceration, bleeding/easy bruising, and, in some individuals, signs of renal compromise, are accounted for cyclooxygenase inhibition in those tissues.

Although renal vascular prostanoids have a role in maintenance of normal renal vascular tone, limitation of their formation by NSAIDs in normal individuals causes no discernible change in renal function. Increased release of renal prostanoids by vasoconstrictors may provide an important mechanism for limitation of vasoconstrictor effects through negative feedback. Thus, in disease or drug-induced states with associated elevations in circulating vasoconstrictors (e.g., congestive heart failure, possibly even diuretic use), or in renal/other diseases where renal production of prostanoids is already subnormal, NSAIDs may be more likely to produce decrements in renal function. Certain of the newer NSAIDs have been reported to have a prostacyclin-sparing effect (ibuprofen, sulindac), which could reduce unwanted renal (and gastric) effects. Significant renal effects have been reported for these drugs also, however.

In contrast to renal effects, gastric effects of NSAIDs are common. Despite some data to indicate that mucosal adaptation may occur on continued administration, complications can be severe. Replacement therapy is one therapeutic option. Two orally effective PGE_1 analogs, misoprostil and rioprostil, have been developed for concomitant use with NSAIDs; PGE_1 analogs are not only preventive, they also appear to accelerate healing of existing lesions. Systemic manifestations of the PGE_1 analogs are minimal, with mild diarrhea somewhat predictably the only frequent side effect. Only misoprostil is currently available in this country.

For completeness of coverage, it should be noted that PGE_2 is thought to mediate temperature elevation subsequent to inflammation or infection, as a mediator for pyrogens (e.g., endogenous pyrogen, IL-1). The antipyretic effects of NSAIDs are thus attributable to decreased formation of PGE_2 in the CNS (hypothalamus). The analgesic effects of NSAIDs are also in part due to inhibition of cyclooxygenase, since inflammatory mediators that cause pain also elicit formation of arachidonic acid metabolites, which then act to enhance the pain effect.

As indicated previously, most cells have an additional pathway for conversion of arachidonic acid, namely the lipoxygenase(s). It has been suggested and partially documented that inhibition of the cyclooxygenase by NSAIDs may result in shunting of arachidonic acid through lipoxygenase, as depicted in Fig. 2-6. The consequences of shunting do not appear to be significant in most individuals in vivo, with some possible exceptions. NSAID hypersensitivity, manifested usually as intense bronchoconstriction and angioneurotic edema, may result from the combination of shunting and unusual production or sensitivity or both to shunt products such as leukotrienes. Shunting through lipoxygenase could also blunt the anti-inflammatory effect of NSAIDs since alternate/additional pro-inflammatory lipoxygenase product mediators would still be formed. This could be of particular significance in that LTB_4 can elicit formation of IL-1, also a mediator of inflammation (see chapter 3). Some side effects, particularly gastrointestinal ones, have also been suggested

Fig. 2-6. Possible scheme for shunting of arachidonic acid (AA) through the (5-) lipoxygenase pathway as a consequence of NSAID inhibition of cylooxygenase (CO)/PGES (prostaglandin endoperoxide synthase). In some individuals, hypersensitivity reactions may be induced/enhanced by this mechanism.

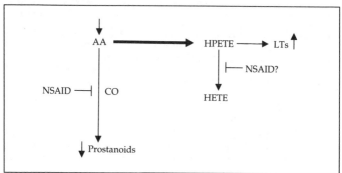

to result from drug-induced imbalance between cyclooxygenase and lipoxygenase products.

In cases where shunting is a suspected contributor to problems, the ideal drug might be one that inhibits both the lipoxygenase(s) and cyclooxygenase (or limits liberation of arachidonic acid; see chapter 3). Such drugs have indeed been sought, and even adequately developed for in vitro use. Lipoxygenase inhibitors generally also have some inhibitory effects on cyclooxygenase, but dose and unwanted effect considerations have been problematic. Thus, clinically useful dual inhibitors have yet to be developed. Indomethacin at high doses has been suggested to inhibit lipoxygenase, and also PLA_2, both of which could account for the greater efficacy of indomethacin in certain inflammation states.

For reference, a listing and some basic pharmacokinetic properties of the currently available NSAIDs are summarized in Table 2-2. Several general properties are worthy of note. As mentioned previously, current NSAIDs are weak organic acids. As for aspirin, absorption is favored by low pH (e.g., in the stomach), which increases the proportion of unionized, membrane-permeant drug. At physiologic pH, the NSAIDs are highly ionized; this is reflected in their small volumes of distribution (V_D), with confinement of the majority of drug to plasma and extracellular fluid. In spite of this, the NSAIDs do partition into synovial fluid, and concentrations that are greater than or equal to 50% of levels in plasma are usually achieved.

Many NSAIDs, with the exception of most of the salicylates (including aspirin, excluding diflunisal), are extensively, i.e., greater than or equal to 90%, bound to plasma proteins (mainly albumin). Even the salicylates are greater than or equal to 80% bound. When used in combination with other highly protein-bound drugs, especially those with a narrow margin of safety, the possibility of clinically relevant pharmacokinetic interactions must be considered.

NSAID elimination occurs by metabolism and excretion. Most NSAIDs undergo a significant degree of metabolism, including conjugation through the carboxyl group. The relatively short half-lives that are observed for many of the NSAIDs in part reflect rapid inactivation by conjugation. Because the NSAIDs undergo hepatic metabolism, potential for interaction with other drugs via hepatic enzyme induction or inhibition exists. Induction of self-metabolism has been suggested to account for the apparent tolerance occasionally seen in patients on long-term aspirin (other NSAID?) therapy.

Parent NSAIDs and metabolites are excreted renally or via bile or both. Probenecid, which interferes with the renal and biliary organic acid secretory mechanism, can lower excretion and increase levels and half-life of some NSAIDs. For those NSAIDs that are secreted into bile, e.g., indomethacin and sulindac, enterohepatic circulation may occur, with prolongation of time of action and intensification of gastrointestinal effects. Fenamates may also undergo some degree of enterohepatic circulation.

Although not all NSAIDs are sufficiently uricosuric (or safe) to warrant their use for that purpose, most NSAIDs do promote significant uric acid excretion (see chapter 5). The uricosuric effect of NSAIDs

Table 2-2. Pharmacokinetic data for anti-inflammatory analgesics

Generic name	Serum half-life (hrs)	Protein binding (%)	V_d (L/kg)	Biotrans-formation	Excretion
Salicylates					
Acetylsalicylic acid (ASA)	0.2	80	0.1–0.35	Hyd Con Oxi	Ren
Sodium salicylate	2–30	80	0.1–0.35	Con Oxi	Ren
Choline salicylate	2–30	80	0.1–0.35	Con Oxi	Ren
Choline magnesium salicylate	2–30	80	0.1–0.35	Con Oxi	Ren
Salicylamide	2			Con Oxi	Ren
Diflunisal	8–12	99	0.09	Con	Ren
Pyrazolones					
Phenylbutazone	36–168	98	0.08	Oxi Con	Ren Bil
Oxyphenbutazone	24–72	98	0.08	Con	Ren Bil
Sulfinpyrazone	3–8	98	0.16	Oxi Con	Ren
Indole/pyrrole acetic acids					
Indomethacin	6–12	90	1.0	Oxi Con	Ren Bil
Sulindac (Indene)	7	93	Not avail.	Oxi Red	Ren Bil
Etodolac	7.3	>99	0.13	Hyx Con	Ren
Tolmetin	1–6	99	0.1	Con Hyx	Ren

21

Table 2-2. Pharmacokinetic data for anti-inflammatory analgesics (cont.)

Generic name	Serum half-life (hrs)	Protein binding (%)	V_d(L/kg)	Biotrans-formation	Excretion
Phenylpropionic acids					
Fenoprofen	2.5	99	0.08	Oxi Con	Ren
Flurbiprofen	4	99	0.1	Oxi Con	Ren
Ibuprofen	2	99	0.12	Oxi Con	Ren Bil
Ketoprofen	1-35	94	0.1	Oxi Con	Ren
Naphthylproprionic acids					
Naproxen	12-15	99	0.1-0.35	Dem	Ren
Naproxen sodium	12-15	99	0.1-0.35	Dem	Ren
Anthranilic acids					
Meclofenamate	4	99	Not avail.	Oxi Con	Ren Bil
Mefenamic acid	4	99	Not avail.	Oxi Hyx	Ren Bil
Diclofenac sodium	1-2	99	0.13	Con	Ren Bil
Oxicam					
Piroxicam	35-45	99	0.12	Hyx Con Hyd	Ren

Key: Con, conjugation; Dem, demethylation; Hyd, hydrolysis; Hyx, hydroxylation; Oxi, oxidation; red, reduction; Bil, biliary.
Source: Modified from H. Kalant and W. Roschlau (eds.). *Principles of Modern Pharmacology* (2nd ed.). Philadelphia: Decker, 1989. P. 325. With permission from The Book Committee, Department of Pharamacology, University of Toronto.

22

is mediated by inhibition of tubular reabsorption of uric acid and occurs predictably for the class of drugs with notable exceptions. One exception is a paradoxical **decrease** in net urate excretion at low doses, particularly for aspirin because of its relatively weak uricosuric potential even at high doses. Because of its weak effects, but high affinity for the binding site, (low dose) aspirin can also effectively antagonize (reduce) the uricosuric effect of other drugs. Another exception may be tolmetin's suggested lack of (significant) uricosuric effects.

Methotrexate, formerly known as amethopterin, is frequently used together with NSAIDs, and a frequently mentioned theoretical result is methotrexate toxicity. The real incidence of NSAID-induced methotrexate toxicity is unclear, however. One mechanism may involve decreased renal elimination of methotrexate, an organic acid, by competition for the transporter by acidic NSAIDs. Another possibility is displacement of methotrexate from protein-binding sites by NSAIDs, resulting in increased free (active) methotrexate.

A number of "idiopathic" interactions have been reported for individual NSAIDs that may or may not be applicable to the class or to structural subclasses. For example, indomethacin antagonizes the antihypertensive effects of beta-blockers, converting enzyme inhibitors, and others. It is unclear whether other NSAIDs act similarly to indomethacin.

Specific NSAID Classes

Salicylates

Acetylsalicylic acid was first synthesized in the mid-1850s and was marketed by Bayer Pharmaceuticals in 1899; it is thus approaching its one hundreth year of open usage. The common name **aspirin** (German: **A**cetyl-**Spir**äe-Säure [acid]) indicates both its chemical nature and the fact that it is related to the salicylates common to *Spirea* species, e.g., willow (bark). The long history of use of the latter, and many other salicylate-containing plants, to treat fever, inflammation, gout, and malaria, among others, provided the impetus for development of aspirin. Aspirin is hydrolyzed in vivo to salicylic acid.

High anti-inflammatory doses, as well as accidental overdoses, of aspirin can result in the syndrome known as **salicylism**. Briefly, depending on the blood levels achieved, the symptoms can include tinnitus, elevated body temperature (secondary to uncoupling of oxidative phosphorylation), and increased (early, lower concentrations) or decreased (later, higher concentrations) respiration, with concomitant respiratory alkalosis or acidosis, respectively. The latter can be worsened by aspirin-induced metabolic acidosis. Two factors contribute significantly to the development of salicylism. The first factor is saturable metabolism of salicylate by hepatic enzymes. The ceiling on metabolic conversion significantly increases the half-life. The metabolic ceiling in fact also increases half-life at anti-inflammatory doses, from the 3–6 hours seen with analgesic/antipyretic doses, to 15–30 hours with anti-inflammatory doses. The second is saturable protein binding for aspirin/salicylates. Thus, sharp increases in free (active) drug with only small increases in dose are possible, especially on acute exposure. Chronic high-dose blood levels may be partially offset by induced metabolism increases.

Aspirin is an effective, albeit not outstanding, inhibitor of cyclo-oxygenase, an attribute that contributes to its anti-inflammatory actions. The nonacetylated salicylates (e.g., sodium, magnesium, choline, and salicyl- salicylates) are ineffective inhibitors of cyclo-oxygenase, although they are modestly anti-inflammatory. Neutrophil inhibitory effects probably contribute to aspirin effects and may be a major component of the effects of the other salicylates. Decreased formation of bradykinin, secondary to aspirin-induced decreases in plasmin, may also enhance anti-inflammatory effectiveness.

The newest of the salicylate-type compounds is diflunisal, a fluorinated aromatic salicylate. Its outstanding feature is its long half-life, which allows for less frequent dosing. Diflunisal is **not** hydrolyzed to salicylate. Like salicylates, however, its excretion (pharmacokinetics) is dose-dependent. The long half-life of diflunisal can result in a long time lag to plateau levels and thus to optimal effect; the lag can be overcome by use of a loading dose.

The side effect incidence with aspirin may be slightly higher than with newer NSAIDs. Worthy of note is the association of aspirin use and occurrence of Reye's syndrome in children: A potential mechanism involves acetylation of mitochondria by aspirin, analogous to aspirin-acetylation of cyclooxygenase.

Pyrazolones

The precursors for this class of compounds were antipyrine and aminopyrine, introduced prior to aspirin in the late 1800s. Though these drugs were quite effective anti-inflammatory (analgesic, antipyretic) agents, occurrence of agranulocytosis subsequent to their use was fairly common. Two additional members of this class of drugs were developed for anti-inflammatory use: phenylbutazone and its active metabolite, oxyphenbutazone. Both compounds have very long half-lives (> 70 hours), which should be noted because of the potential for drug accumulation. Unfortunately, the offspring agents produce excellent anti-inflammatory (and uricosuric) effects but are at least as toxic as the parent compounds. In addition to all the "usual" unwanted NSAID effects, the list of potentially serious and even fatal hematologic disturbances attributable to the pyrazolones includes leukopenia, agranulocytosis, aplastic anemia, and even leukemia. The mechanism(s) for the hematologic effects is unclear. A third compound, sulfinpyrazone, was developed primarily for uricosuric effects (see chapter 5) and is without significant anti-inflammatory activity.

Indole/Indene- and Pyrrole Acetic Acids

Serotonin, or 5-hydroxytryptamine (5-HT), and its amino acid precursor, tryptophan, were proposed at one time as mediators of inflammation in humans, based on data for various animals. Because 5-HT is an indole, indoles with **anti**-inflammatory activity were sought and indomethacin was identified. Indomethacin is a very effective anti-inflammatory agent but produces use-limiting CNS side effects in addition to all the usual NSAID side effects. Because 5-HT is involved in the etiology of migraine headache, it has been suggested that indomethacin's structural similarity to 5-HT may somehow account for its ability to produce intense headache, and other CNS effects, in a significant number of people who take it.

Sulindac is structurally related to indomethacin. Sulindac itself is inactive and must be converted to an active sulfide metabolite in vivo; formation of nonactive metabolites occurs simultaneously. Sulindac, on introduction, was stated to produce significantly fewer side effects than indomethacin. Although the incidence may be lower and the intensity less, the range is the same and includes CNS effects.

Tolmetin and zomepirac are closely related to indomethacin and sulindac: The structures contain a pyrrole ring. Zomepirac was withdrawn from the market several years ago, subsequent to occurrence of severe adverse effects. Tolmetin is a very effective anti-inflammatory compound, with significant side effect occurrence, including some in the CNS. The incidence and severity are reportedly less than with indomethacin and possibly as low as with the phenylpropionic acids.

A new market addition to this group is etodolac (Lodine). Its half-life approximates those of other members of the group (6.0–7.5 hours). The most notable feature is a low occurrence of gastrointestinal symptoms, reportedly not significantly greater than those with placebo.

Phenylpropionic Acids

The first approved and marketed member of this group was ibuprofen. A notable characteristic of ibuprofen, and many other members of the group, is somewhat greater tolerance than for other NSAID groups. Indeed, the tolerance and safety records for prescription ibuprofen contributed to its eventual release as an over-the-counter drug, albeit in lower-dose preparations (200 mg). Ibuprofen, and possibly others of the group, are sporadically reported to have a sparing effect on prostacyclin production in vivo, which could account in part for the relative lack of serious side effects. All the members of the group have useful anti-inflammatory effects, and partition into synovial fluid. No outstanding differences exist among the drugs in the group, although several individual properties are worthy of note.

The anti-inflammatory effects of flurbiprofen are somewhat greater than those of ibuprofen and, indeed, may equal indomethacin. Flurbiprofen side effects may be somewhat more intense and frequent than for other members of the class. Carprofen, a possible new approval in this class, has excellent anti-inflammatory properties, is relatively lipophilic, partitions well into synovial fluid, and has a half-life (13–27 hours) that makes it usable on a twice per day schedule.

Most members of this group are completely absorbed after oral administration, and absorption is not affected by food intake; however, fenoprofen absorption can be incomplete and also limited by food intake.

Naproxen has a relatively long half-life and can be used twice per day. Toxicity (side effects) may in part be limited by plasma protein binding such that blood levels cannot exceed a limit regardless of dose. The absorption of naproxen can be delayed by food as well as by antacids (magnesium oxide as well as aluminum hydroxide types); however, these effects on naproxen absorption are stated to be insignificant.

The half-life of ketoprofen, in contrast to most other members of this group, can be greater than a day or as short as an hour. The mechanism(s) accounting for the variability is unknown.

Fenamates (Anthranilates)

Although there are two fenamates in this group, mefenamic acid is not used for its anti-inflammatory activity. Meclofenamic acid (sodium) is a very effective inhibitor of cyclooxygenase, and direct antagonism of prostanoid effects has also been suggested. This drug produces significant gastrointestinal effects, perhaps in part because of enterohepatic circulation.

Diclofenac also belongs to the general group of anthranilate NSAIDs, although it has an acetic acid substitution rather than the simple carboxyl of the true fenamates. Its advantages may be a reduced incidence and severity of side effects. Its absorption may be delayed (but not prevented) by food intake. In addition, the drug undergoes significant first-pass metabolism: Hepatic dysfunction could increase expected drug levels relative to dose administered.

Piroxicam

The long half-life (**average** ≈ 50 hours) allows for once a day dosing; however, it should be remembered that accumulation occurs as a result, and steady state levels are not reached for four to five half-lives (anywhere from one to two weeks to > three weeks). The side effects associated with this drug can be severe and include some CNS effects (e.g., headache) in addition to common NSAID effects.

Clinical Indications

Some of the most widely used (in the United States) salicylate preparations are listed in Table 2-3, and all of the currently available (in the United States) nonsalicylate NSAIDs are listed in Table 2-4. Of the nonsalicylate NSAIDs, only ibuprofen is currently available without prescription. It is marketed in 200-mg tablets as an analgesic under a number of different trade names (e.g., Nuprin, Advil). Of the three major pharmacologic actions of the NSAIDs (antipyretic, analgesic, anti-inflammatory), the most interesting in the management of rheumatic disease patients is the anti-inflammatory effect, though these agents are widely used as analgesics. In fact, along with acetaminophen, they are the only class of non-narcotic analgesics available in this country. In the rheumatic diseases, fever is usually a manifestation of a serious exacerbation requiring more intensive therapy than the NSAIDs, or it is a manifestation of a concomitant infection requiring precise diagnosis; consequently the antipyretic effect of these drugs is seldom a clinical indication for their use. In fact, their ability to mask fever might be considered

Table 2-3. Some commonly used salicylate preparations available in the United States

Aspirin

Trade name	Preparation
Easprin (by prescription)	Enteric-coated, delayed-release, 975-mg ASA
Zorprin (by prescription)	Enteric-coated "zero-order release," 800-mg ASA
Alka-Seltzer	Sodium bicarbonate and citric acid with 325-mg ASA
Anacin	Caffeine 32-mg with 400- or 500-mg ASA
Arthritis Pain Formula	Buffered, 486-mg ASA
Ascriptin	150- or 300-mg of mg-al hydroxide with 325-mg ASA
Bayer	325-mg or 650-mg ("time-release") ASA
Bufferin	325- or 486-mg of ASA with buffers
Cama	600-mg ASA with mg-al hydroxide
Ecotrin	Enteric-coated 325- or 500-mg ASA
Encaprin	325- or 500-mg ASA
Excedrin	Acetaminophen, 97 mg Salicylamide, 130 mg Caffeine, 65 mg ASA, 194 mg
Goody's Powders	Acetaminophen, 260 mg Caffeine, 32 mg ASA, 520 mg
Stanback Powders	Salicylamide, 200 mg Caffeine, 15 mg ASA, 650 mg
Vanquish	Acetaminophen, 194 mg Caffeine, 33 mg Mg-al hydroxide ASA, 227 mg

Nonacetylated salicylates (by prescription)

Generic name	Trade name	Tablet size (mg)
Choline magnesium trisalicylate	Trilisate	500 750 1000
Magnesium salicylate	Magan	500
Salsalate	Disalcid	500 750
	Persisten	486, with 162 ASA
	Salflex	500 750
Sodium salicylate	Pabalate	300, with 300 of sodium aminobenzoate

Key: ASA, acetylsalicylic acid; mg-al, magnesium-aluminum.

Table 2-4. Prescription nonsalicylate NSAIDs available in the United States

Generic name	Trade name	Capsule/tablet size	Usual anti-inflammatory dosage
Phenylbutazone*	Butazoilidin	100 mg	100 mg tid–qid
Indomethacin*	Indocin	25 mg 50 mg 75 mg (sustained release)	25–50 mg tid–qid
Mefenamic acid	Ponstel (sold as an analgesic)	250 mg	250 mg q6h
Ibuprofen*	Motrin Rufen	300 mg 400 mg 600 mg 800 mg	300–800 mg qid
Fenoprofen calcium*	Nalfon	300 mg 600 mg	300–600 mg qid
Naproxen	Naprosyn	250 mg 375 mg 500 mg	250–500 mg bid
	Anaprox (sold as an analgesic)	275 mg 550 mg	275–550 mg bid
Tolmetin sodium	Tolectin	200 mg 400 mg 600 mg	400 mg tid–qid
Sulindac*	Clinoril	150 mg 200 mg	150–200 mg bid
Meclofenamate*	Meclomen	50 mg 100 mg	50–100 mg tid–qid
Piroxicam	Feldene	10 mg 20 mg	10–20 mg once a day
Diflunisal	Dolobid	250 mg 500 mg	250–500 mg q8–12h
Ketoprofen	Orudis	25 mg 50 mg 75 mg	50–75 mg tid–qid
Diclofenac	Voltaren	25 mg 50 mg 75 mg	50 mg qid–75 mg bid
Flurbiprofen	Ansaid	50 mg 100 mg	100 mg bid–tid
Ketorolac tromethamine	Toradol (sold as parenteral analgesic)	15 mg/cc 30 mg/cc	15–60 mg IM as analgesic
Etodolac	Lodine	200 mg 300 mg	200 mg bid to 300 mg qid

*Available generically.

an unwanted effect. In the following paragraphs, analgesia will be considered briefly and modification of the inflammatory response discussed in more detail.

ANALGESIC ACTION

In equivalent doses the analgesic effects of the NSAIDs are roughly equal, and the dose required for an analgesic effect is less than that required for an anti-inflammatory action. Approximately 650 mg of aspirin, 400 mg of ibuprofen, 650 mg of acetaminophen, and 30 mg of codeine appear to be equivalent in terms of analgesia. For aspirin, at least, no evidence shows that doses in excess of 650 mg provide additional analgesic effect. Maximally effective analgesic doses of the other NSAIDs are less certain. The analgesic effect of the NSAIDs is qualitatively different from that of the narcotics; the NSAIDs are more effective for the pain of musculoskeletal inflammation and trauma, dental pain, and the pain of serositis than they are for visceral or neuropathic pain. Consequently they are relatively ideal analgesics for most rheumatic pain problems; however, most rheumatic pain problems represent indications for regular anti-inflammatory dosages of the NSAIDs. The efficacy and safety of using analgesic doses of one NSAID in a patient taking anti-inflammatory doses of another have not been established and remain quite doubtful. This practice is usually not recommended. Therefore codeine and other minor narcotics and acetaminophen are usually prescribed for prn use in patients taking anti-inflammatory doses of NSAIDs.

In practice NSAIDs are commonly prescribed for painful conditions not known to be associated with inflammation, and taken together these conditions may account for the majority of NSAID prescriptions written in this country. In addition to ill-defined and undiagnosed pain syndromes, these conditions commonly include low back pain, axial degenerative joint disease, local myofascial pain syndromes, and the syndrome of fibromyalgia (or fibrositis). If any benefits are derived from this practice, they must be attributed to the analgesic effect of these agents or to a placebo effect, very often the latter. Considering the potential toxicity of NSAIDs, it can be strongly recommended that only analgesic doses be used in these circumstances, and even then with extreme caution in those at high risk for side effects, such as the elderly population.

Many of the nonsalicylate NSAIDs have not been approved by the FDA for use as analgesics, and even when they have been approved for analgesia, the recommended dose may be in excess of that required for this action. Currently mefenamic acid, ibuprofen, fenoprofen, naproxen (Anaprox), diflunisal, ketoprofen, ketorolac, and etodolac are approved for use in mild to moderate pain. For some of these agents, the manufacturer's recommended analgesic dose is as great as or actually exceeds the recommended anti-inflammatory dose. Little evidence suggests that this is necessary, and lower doses are advised especially if the drug is to be used regularly. For only occasional use, the larger doses are probably safe, even if unnecessary.

ANTI-INFLAMMATORY ACTION

The most common rheumatic anti-inflammatory indications for the NSAIDs are listed in Table 2-5. Almost all of the NSAIDs are approved for use in rheumatoid arthritis and osteoarthritis, and several are approved for use in gout, ankylosing spondylitis, and acute tendinitis and bursitis. FDA approval simply reflects the focus of pre- and postmarketing clinical trials and in no way indicates the true efficacy of the drug in any rheumatic disease. FDA approval also has not significantly impacted on patterns of usage, except perhaps in children. Nine common questions concerning the anti-inflammatory use of these agents are summarized in Table 2-6. Each will be addressed individually.

Dose

Even in their maximally tolerated doses, the NSAIDs uncommonly abolish all signs and symptoms of the disorder being treated. For a few of the agents experimental evidence exists for a linear relationship between anti-inflammatory effect and blood level (or dose), and this relationship is widely assumed to be true for all of them. For the salicylates, blood levels are available and therapeutic and toxic ranges can be determined accurately; for the other NSAIDs, one must rely on the manufacturer's dose recommendations. Therefore, it seems reasonable to adjust salicylate dose according to blood level and to use maximum recommended doses of the other agents, taking patient size and age into consideration (see Table 2-4 for maximum recommended doses). This approach would allow for an early determination of efficacy but would also maximize early side effects. Alternatively, for the nonsalicylate NSAIDs, one could begin with a smaller dose and gradually increase it toward the maximum according to clinical response, but these dose adjustments may require several weeks. Whatever the approach, true effectiveness can seldom be determined until a maximum dose has been given.

Table 2-5. Common indications for NSAID anti-inflammatory dosages

Active rheumatoid arthritis
Arthritis and serositis of systemic lupus erythematosus
Arthritis of the scleroderma syndromes
Arthritis of Sjögren's syndrome
Arthritis and serositis of mixed connective tissue disease
Osteoarthritis with an inflammatory component (primarily hip)
Active ankylosing spondylitis
Reiter's syndrome
Active psoriatic arthritis
Acute gouty arthritis
Acute pseudogout
Acute bursitis, tendinitis, or tenosynovitis
Arthritis of hypersensitivity vasculitis
Systemic-onset juvenile rheumatoid arthritis*
Polyarticular juvenile rheumatoid arthritis*
Pauciarticular juvenile rheumatoid arthritis*

*Of the nonsalicylate NSAIDs, only naproxen and tolmetin are approved for use in children.

Regular Use

In the premarketing clinical trials of all of the NSAIDs, anti-inflammatory effectiveness was determined on the basis of regular use, presumably reflected by relatively stable blood levels. Furthermore it makes no clinical sense to intermittently suppress an inflammatory response. Consequently patients should clearly understand that their NSAID prescription is for regular use as long as clinical evidence exists of a persisting inflammatory process.

Effectiveness

In clinical trials rheumatoid arthritis has been the most common human model of inflammation studied, and it is relatively ideal for this purpose since its inflammatory response is so readily apparent and easy to measure. The effects that have been most often sought are symptomatic improvement (less pain, stiffness, and fatigue) and less joint inflammation (swelling and tenderness). Since NSAIDs seldom completely abolish all signs and symptoms of the inflammatory process, the patient and the physician must agree on what is a satisfactory response. In making such a determination, the patient will usually focus on symptoms; consequently the physician might wish to focus on signs.

Best NSAID

The best NSAID is the one that works best for the individual patient's individual problem. Considerable experimental and some clinical evidence exists that phenylbutazone and indomethacin are the most potent NSAIDs, but the former is widely regarded as too toxic for almost any use, and the latter is clearly associated with more side effects than any of the remaining ones. Otherwise there seem to be no major differences in effectiveness of equivalent doses among the other NSAIDs, including the salicylates. In the clinical trials, almost all of the newer NSAIDs have been about as effective as full therapeutic doses of aspirin, but these trials have predominantly involved patients with rheumatoid arthritis and osteoarthritis. Some evidence and considerable clinical experience suggest that indomethacin is more effective in certain diseases than are the

Table 2-6. Nine most commonly asked questions concerning the anti-inflammatory effect of the NSAIDs

1. What dose is required?
2. Is regular use necessary?
3. How is effectiveness determined?
4. Is one (or some) drug(s) better than the others? (*or* which is the best?)
5. Will one NSAID work when (several) others have not? (*or* do some patients respond better to one drug than to others?)
6. How long should one drug be tried before it is judged ineffective?
7. Is the effectiveness of an initially successful drug lost with time and continued use?
8. Do NSAIDs alter the course of the disease process being treated?
9. Are combinations of two or more different NSAIDs more effective than one alone?

other NSAIDs. In acute crystal-induced arthritis and in the spondyloarthropathies, salicylates are relatively ineffective, and indomethacin often seems to be superior to the other NSAIDs—when it is tolerated. Indomethacin may also be superior in the management of serositis, osteoarthritis of the hip, and acute bursitis-tendinitis. Because of its side effects, indomethacin would not be a wise choice for rheumatoid arthritis unless the less toxic NSAIDs had failed. There are too few comparative studies to suggest the superiority of any one or one class of NSAID in that disease, but surveys have indicated that the salicylates are the most widely used agents among rheumatologists. For most clinical situations, including rheumatoid arthritis, considerations other than efficacy usually determine the choice of an NSAID preparation; these considerations include physician and patient preference, expense, convenience of dosage schedule, and side effects.

Selective Response

Few prospective studies clearly indicate that individual patients may respond to one NSAID when they have not responded to others, but clinical experience has suggested that this is true. Some physicians even provide their patients with three or more different drugs to try sequentially, allowing the patient to decide which is best. It has been suggested that agents from different classes be tried under these circumstances; for example, if a patient has not responded to an arylpropionic acid (e.g., ibuprofen), an indole acetic acid (sulindac) might be substituted. In clinical practice these sequential trials often have more to do with side effects than with efficacy.

Duration of Trial

Onset of NSAID action is rapid and the anti-inflammatory effect usually becomes apparent within a few half-lives of the drug; however, most controlled clinical trials have extended beyond two weeks and most for a month or longer. In some of the more protracted studies, evidence exists for accruing benefits after a month or longer of continued therapy, but the most impressive responses have usually been in the first two weeks. Consequently two- to four-week trials can be recommended; no response at two weeks justifies discontinuing the agent, whereas a partial or equivocal response indicates an additional two-week trial.

Loss of Efficacy

Several uncontrolled and unblinded observations suggest that the NSAID being investigated continued to be effective over a year or longer of continuous use, and no published data indicate that secondary failures occur; therefore, the question of "immunity" so often raised by patients is not a recognized phenomenon. It is likely that clinical worsening in the face of a NSAID that has apparently been effective for months or years represents a fundamental change in the disease process and not in the efficacy of the drug. In practice, however, it is usually necessary to handle this situation as one would a primary failure in order to prove that it is the disease and not the response to the drug that is changing.

Disease Modification

Disease modification by any class of antirheumatic drug is a very difficult action to prove, and even a suggestion of disease-modifying effect requires controlled studies extending beyond the period of a year. Furthermore the question of what constitutes a disease-modifying action must be addressed. In rheumatoid arthritis halting or slowing progression of joint destruction as evidenced by joint roentgenography has been considered a disease-modifying effect, and preliminary evidence exists that at least one NSAID (etodolac) may do this. In general, however, the NSAIDs are not regarded as disease-modifying agents, though very few studies have even attempted to test for this action. As yet no indication exists for continuing NSAID therapy after the inflammatory process is arrested by other agents or remits spontaneously.

Combinations of NSAIDs

Side effects severely limit any consideration of using combinations of full therapeutic doses of two or more different NSAIDs together, and this issue has rarely been addressed in controlled clinical trials. In one study anti-inflammatory doses of naproxen and choline magnesium trisalicylate together were marginally more effective than either drug alone, but a clinically important additive or synergistic effect was not demonstrated. Any marginal benefit that might result from combination NSAID therapy does not warrant the risk of additional side effects and the expense that would result; therefore, this practice cannot be recommended.

A SPECIAL COMMENT ON THE SALICYLATES

Only drugs hydrolyzed to salicylic acid, the active metabolite, will be considered salicylates; therefore, diflunisal, a difluorophenyl derivative of salicylic acid, does not qualify. Aspirin differs from the nonacetylated salicylates in its ability to irreversibly acetylate certain proteins, most notably cyclooxygenase. This action does not appear to play a major role in its anti-inflammatory effect and will not be addressed further in this chapter. Slight variations exist among the salicylates in terms of available salicylic acid, but these differences are not clinically important, and dosages will be discussed as if all of the salicylates were equivalent. In equivalent (or the same) doses or using comparable blood salicylate levels, no significant difference appears in the anti-inflammatory effect of aspirin and the nonacetylated salicylates; consequently, they can be used interchangeably.

A minimum anti-inflammatory blood salicylate level is 15 mg/dl, and toxicity begins to appear with levels greater than 35 mg/dl; therefore, an acceptable therapeutic range is between 15 mg/dl and 35 mg/dl. The dosage required to produce this range is notoriously variable. In adults it ranges from less than 3 to greater than 6 gm/day. There is increasing evidence in patients with rheumatoid arthritis, at least, that ototoxicity is not a reliable indicator of blood salicylate level. Up to 30% of patients will become symptomatic at subtherapeutic levels, and a smaller number will attain toxic levels without symptoms; in fact, ototoxicity at subtherapeutic levels may be the most common reason for having to abandon salicylates in favor of some other NSAID. Ototoxicity is especially unreliable in patients with known hearing deficits and in the older population. It is recommended for the average adult that salicylates be started in dosages of about 3 gm/day. If no side effects appear after about a week, the dosage can be increased to 4 gm/day. Above 4 gm/day, dosage increments should probably be monitored by measuring blood salicylate levels.

Because of their relatively peculiar excretion kinetics, once a therapeutic level has been achieved, salicylates can usually be given daily in two divided doses about 12 hours apart with acceptable fluctuations in blood salicylate levels. Adequate clinical studies of the nonacetylated salicylates and enteric-coated aspirin support the acceptability of this twice-daily schedule, and only enteric-coated aspirin will be recommended in anti-inflammatory doses (see Clinical Aspects of Side Effects). Since there is rarely any urgency in achieving a steady state salicylate level, twice a day dosage schedules can generally be suggested from the onset of therapy. Consequently salicylates share with some of the nonsalicylate NSAIDs a convenient dosage schedule, which is appreciated by many patients. The same excretion kinetics that allow for this practice predispose to serious toxicity if significant amounts of additional salicylate are added to a therapeutic blood level; therefore, these patients should be warned not to take additional salicylate-containing preparations on their own.

Many clinicians, including some rheumatologists, feel that salicylates have been outmoded by the newer nonsalicylate NSAIDs, and nonsalicylate NSAIDs are clearly preferable in some situations (e.g., spondyloarthropathies and gout). In most situations involving clinical inflammation, however, the newer agents have no discernable advantages in terms of efficacy, and many of the side effects can be minimized by the appropriate choice of salicylate preparation (see next section). Considering efficacy, convenience, toxicity, and expense, the salicylates would seem to be a reasonable first choice in most clinical situations when a NSAID is genuinely indicated.

Clinical Aspects of Side Effects

For most of the NSAIDs requiring a prescription, the side effects reported by the manufacturer primarily reflect those detected during the premarketing studies of the agent, and these studies typically involved subjects at relatively low risk for toxicity. For most such studies, the elderly and patients with known renal, liver, and gastrointestinal diseases were excluded. Much of the postmarketing toxicity reported in the literature reflects side effects observed in these high-risk patients, and these side effects may not be accurately represented in the drug's package insert (or in the *Physician's Desk Reference*). Not all of the side effects discussed here have been reported for all of the NSAIDs, and distinctions among them, when appropriate, will be made; however, it seems likely that all of these agents have at least the potential to produce almost all of the side effects reported for one or a limited number. Major NSAID side effects are summarized in Table 2-7. Relative frequencies are based on averages reported in the package inserts or in the published literature, or both. Each of these side effects will be discussed individually in the following paragraphs.

OTOTOXICITY

Symptoms of ototoxicity are reported commonly by patients taking diflunisal and the salicylates and uncommonly by patients taking the other NSAIDs. The usual symptoms are tinnitus, hearing loss, or other unusual sensations in the ear such as a "stuffy feeling."

Table 2-7. Major side effects of the NSAIDs

Side effect	Estimated frequency*	Comment
Ototoxicity	Common	Very common with salicylates and diflunisal; uncommon with other agents.
Hypersensitivity	Uncommon	Primarily asthma or urticaria, or both; circulatory collapse rare. May be less likely with nonacetylated salicylates.
Cutaneous	Common	Pruritus and nonspecific rashes. Commonly reported; often unrelated to the NSAID.
Hepatic	Uncommon	Most often mild asymptomatic elevations of one or more hepatic enzymes.
CNS	Uncommon	Uncommon with most NSAIDs but common with indomethacin. Cognitive dysfunction may be common in the elderly.
Renal		
Due to prostaglandin inhibition	Uncommon	Uncommon in low-risk patients; common in those with edema states and renal insufficiency. Hyperkalemia and renal failure of most concern.
Idiosyncratic	Rare	Interstitial nephritis or nephrotic syndrome; may be most often seen with indomethacin, or fenoprofen.
Gastrointestinal		
Upper and lower GI symptoms	Very common	Correlate poorly with bleeding and demonstrable lesions.
Gastric erosions, ulcerations	Very common	May be less common with nonacetylated salicylates or enteric-coated aspirin.
Small-bowel and colonic lesions	Rare	Relationship of NSAIDs and peptic duodenal ulcer disease unclear.

*Very common = > 10%
Common   = 5–10%
Uncommon   = 1–4%
Rare   = < 1%

Clearly the salicylates (and diflunisal) can cause these symptoms; it is less clear that the other NSAIDs do. Intermittent tinnitus is very common in the general population and is most often unrelated to any drug therapy, so coincidental associations probably occur commonly. When the symptoms are drug induced, they are completely reversible on its withdrawal; no permanent residuals remain.

The major problem with salicylate ototoxicity is that it limits the use of these drugs in a significant proportion of the population. As many as 30% of patients with rheumatoid arthritis develop symptoms of ototoxicity on subtherapeutic salicylate doses, and few are willing to tolerate worsening symptoms in order to achieve a therapeutic level. Because of the effects of the disease on the ear, patients with rheumatoid arthritis may be more susceptible to this effect than are other patients.

HYPERSENSITIVITY

A portion of the population, perhaps 1–2%, are unusually sensitive to the inhibitory effects of the NSAIDs on the cyclooxygenase and lipooxygenase enzyme systems and will develop symptoms on exposure to almost any of the NSAIDs. These symptoms usually consist of asthma, urticaria, or both, but fully developed anaphylactoid reactions may occur. Although hypersensitivity is not confined to patients with the triad of vasomotor rhinitis, nasal polyposis, and asthma, patients with this syndrome appear to be much more susceptible. In fact, a number of patients with asthma alone will experience worsening bronchospasm on exposure to a NSAID. The more potent inhibitors of cyclooxygenase, such as indomethacin, may be the worst offenders; the weak inhibitors, especially the nonacetylated salicylates, may be the least likely to cause a hypersensitivity reaction; however, with a history of an anaphylactoid reaction to any NSAID, extreme caution is recommended in prescribing any other, even very low doses of nonacetylated salicylate. If the drug must be given, it should be administered first in a controlled environment with resuscitative equipment and drugs available.

CUTANEOUS REACTIONS

Pruritus and minor rashes are commonly reported by patients taking NSAIDs, but a causal relationship is frequently difficult to establish. Serious cutaneous reactions are rarely reported. A photosensitizing effect has been most strongly suggested for piroxicam; otherwise phenylbutazone, sulindac, and meclofenamate may have caused more cutaneous reactions than the other available NSAIDs; and phenylbutazone has probably been associated with more severe skin reactions than have the others. Reports have implicated almost all of the NSAIDs (including the salicylates) in isolated cases of erythema nodosum, erythema multiforme (including Stevens-Johnson syndrome), hypersensitivity vasculitis, exfoliative dermatitis, and fixed drug eruptions. For the minor reactions, temporary withdrawal and then reinstitution of the NSAID will help establish a causal relationship. For the more serious reactions, permanent avoidance of that chemical class of NSAID would be prudent.

HEPATIC REACTIONS

Between 1 and 4% of patients taking a NSAID will experience often transient and most often minor elevations of one or more hepatic enzymes; this figure may exceed 5% for aspirin and the reaction may be more serious with diclofenac than with any of the other nonsalicylate NSAIDs. A causal relationship may be difficult to establish since some of the diseases being treated (e.g., rheumatoid arthritis and systemic lupus erythematosus) are themselves associated with occasional hepatic enzyme abnormalities. It is widely thought that children with one of the juvenile arthritis syndromes, adults with rheumatoid arthritis or systemic lupus, patients with prior liver disease, and the elderly are more susceptible to this reaction. Serious hepatic toxicity has rarely been reported and has most often been associated with phenylbutazone, though isolated cases with other agents have also been observed. Should hepatic enzymes be monitored routinely in patients taking these agents regularly? Minor elevations frequently resolve even though the drug is continued, and marked elevations have occasionally been reported to appear suddenly so that their onset would likely have been missed by periodic monitoring. Although the manufacturers of some agents recommend routine testing, the utility of this practice will be difficult to establish; cautious use of these agents in the elderly and in those with prior liver disease can be recommended, however.

CNS REACTIONS

The most common CNS NSAID reaction is severe headache, by far most often occurring with indomethacin. The headache is frequently accompanied by other CNS symptoms, such as dizziness, hallucinations, confusion, depression, and depersonalization reactions. Seizures have also been reported. This reaction usually appears within the first few days of beginning therapy but may also occur after long-term regular use. It responds rapidly to discontinuing the agent. A second type of reaction has been reported in the elderly, so far with only a few of the NSAIDs, but it probably should be expected to occur with all of them. This reaction consists primarily of cognitive dysfunction, often associated with confusion, personality change, depression, and sleeplessness. Simple forgetfulness is often the first symptom. The syndrome usually resolves within a few days of withdrawing the drug. A third CNS reaction has been reported rarely and then primarily in the context of an underlying connective tissue disease. The syndrome is the rapid onset of symptomatic aseptic meningitis, often following the ingestion of a single dose of the drug. It resolves, without other therapy, within 48 hours of discontinuing the NSAID. Ibuprofen, tolmetin, and sulindac have been reported to cause this dramatic reaction.

RENAL REACTIONS

Three different renal side effects of the NSAIDs have been reported: those related to inhibition of renal prostaglandin production (perhaps including edema and elevated blood pressure), a group of idiosyncratic reactions involving interstitial nephritis and the nephrotic syndrome, and those that result from the uricosuric effect of some of the NSAIDs. The most common of these reactions results from renal cyclooxygenase inhibition and is to some degree avoidable since it predominates in patients with underlying renal disease and edema states, conditions in which the NSAIDs should be used with extreme caution, if at all. Specifically the major risk factors for this group of reactions are renal insufficiency or renal failure of any cause; nephrotic syndrome; cirrhosis with edema; heart failure with edema; diabetes mellitus; and the concomitant use of beta-blockers, angiotensin-converting enzyme inhibitors, and potassium-sparing diuretics.

Clinically the three major effects observed are fluid retention (with or without worsening hypertension or heart failure), new or worsened renal insufficiency (occasionally acute renal failure), and hyperkalemia. Whether or not the fluid retention is solely due to inhibition of renal prostaglandin synthesis is open to question since it commonly occurs in subjects with none of the risk factors mentioned previously, and pre-existing hypertension may be worsened in patients with none of these risk factors. Edema alone is often a trivial problem and may be accepted by the patient or managed with low doses of diuretics. Renal insufficiency is widely regarded as an indication for discontinuing the offending NSAID, and hyperkalemia is clearly an indication for such an action since it may reach life-threatening proportions.

Renal insufficiency/failure and hyperkalemia usually occur within a few days of beginning the drug and have been reported most often with indomethacin, especially in the relatively large doses used to treat acute gout. It has been suggested that sulindac may not result in these side effects since its cyclooxygenase-inhibiting metabolite is inactivated in the kidney, but more recent studies do not support this "renal-sparing" effect. It is likely that the nonacetylated salicylates do have a renal-sparing effect because they are weak cyclooxygenase inhibitors, but their safety under these circumstances has not been established. Until or unless the nonacetylated salicylates are proven safe in patients with risk factors for these side effects, all NSAIDs are best avoided in patients with significant renal disease or edema states. This implies that renal function status should be known before a NSAID is prescribed. Otherwise, for patients with diabetes mellitus, for patients at risk because of the drugs listed previously, and for the elderly, a prudent approach would be to recheck the creatinine and electrolytes five to seven days after beginning NSAID therapy.

The rare idiosyncratic reactions of the nephrotic syndrome and interstitial nephritis are not predictable and cannot be avoided, but this type of reaction should be promptly recognized for what it is in any patient with a suggestive clinical picture who is taking a NSAID on a regular basis. Most reports have emphasized the syndrome of acute interstitial nephritis, which is often associated with fever and other systemic features and most often reported with fenoprofen. Perhaps closely related to this syndrome have been the occasional reports of papillary necrosis in patients taking NSAIDs, but a causal relationship has not been established clearly in human subjects.

The uricosuric effect of the NSAIDs is probably of no clinical importance unless the patient has gout or uric acid–related nephrolithiasis. It would be wise to avoid the uricosuric NSAIDs in patients with gout and in those with kidney stones, unless the stones have been documented to be unrelated to uric acid. The hypouricemia achieved with full therapeutic doses of some of these drugs is often impressive though of no significance clinically.

GASTROINTESTINAL SIDE EFFECTS

The most common and the most important NSAID side effects are those affecting the gastrointestinal tract, especially the stomach. They can be viewed from four aspects: symptoms of abdominal pain, dyspepsia, and nausea; acute and severe episodes (predominantly upper gastrointestinal bleeding); subclinical (occult) gastrointestinal blood loss; and endoscopically demonstrated gastrointestinal lesions. The first of these manifestations correlates poorly with the other three, leaving the clinician uncertain as to how seriously symptoms of abdominal pain and nausea should be taken. These complaints are very common with all of the NSAIDs but do not necessarily suggest serious pathology. Conversely the majority of patients presenting with acute and serious pathology (largely bleeding gastric erosions or ulcers) will have had no significant antecedent symptoms; however, the correlation between symptoms and potentially serious pathology is only weak, not absent, so that some effort to exclude upper gastrointestinal bleeding, at least, is warranted in patients with persisting complaints. Otherwise, significant symptoms can be managed by attempting to find a less offensive preparation; indomethacin and phenylbutazone may be the most offensive whereas nonacetylated salicylates and enteric-coated aspirin may be the least. Or symptomatic therapy, usually antacids, might be offered.

Probably the most illuminating technique for identifying potentially serious lesions is endoscopy. Numerous endoscopy studies involving subjects taking NSAIDs on a regular basis over varying periods have lead to the concept of NSAID gastropathy. The pathogenesis of NSAID gastropathy involves inhibition of gastric prostaglandin synthesis leading to the breakdown of a complex mechanism called **gastric cytoprotection**. The loss of cytoprotection results in the gastric erosions and ulcerations seen with the endoscope. NSAID gastropathy differs from peptic ulcer disease in the following ways: Acid does not play the major role (cytoprotection does); the **gastric** mucosa is predominantly affected, the elderly, especially women, seem most susceptible; and the H_2-blocking agents may not be very effective prophylaxis. The stomach has been the major focus of most studies addressing the issue of NSAID-related mucosal injury, but it is now clear that the duodenum is also affected, and it is also clear that NSAIDs will interfere with the healing of pre-existing duodenal ulcer disease or esophagitis.

Controlled and uncontrolled endoscopy studies suggest an alarming prevalence of NSAID-induced mucosal injury. Wide variations exist depending on the particular preparation and the duration of therapy, but up to 20% of regular NSAID users can be expected to have an ulcer and an additional 20–40% can be expected to have erosions without frank ulceration. How often these lesions are complicated by major bleeding or perforation is another question. Although not well documented, occult blood loss must be common; it is thought to make a significant contribution to the anemia so commonly associated with rheumatoid arthritis. On the other hand, studies have suggested that positive tests for occult stool blood in regular NSAID users are often associated with unrelated lesions, suggesting the need for a complete evaluation when positive tests are encountered. The cost effectiveness of this approach is yet another question. In terms of more serious complications of NSAID-induced mucosal injury, 1–4% of regular users will require hospitalization for perforation or bleeding, usually the latter, during each year of therapy. In the elderly and in the debilitated, the mortality of these serious complications is significant. These figures have cast a pall over the long-term and regular use of these agents.

Significant differences may exist among the NSAIDs in terms of their ability to induce mucosal injury, and it seems that full anti-inflammatory doses of most agents are more likely to cause erosions and ulcerations than are smaller analgesic doses. As a strong cyclooxygenase inhibitor, indomethacin should be among the worst offenders, but it is difficult to prove that from existing endoscopy studies. Aspirin in any form that is not enteric coated has been the leading offender in a number of comparative endoscopy studies; enteric-coated aspirin and the nonacetylated salicylates especially the latter are beginning to appear as the least offensive agents. Also, evidence exists that diflunisal and sulindac may cause less mucosal injury than do many of the other agents. Otherwise it is difficult to establish a rank order for the other NSAIDs because of differences in design from one study to another, with the major variations in dosage and duration of therapy.

It may be possible to pharmacologically restore gastric cytoprotection. Conflicting data exist for a protective effect of the H_2-blockers. Though they may help prevent the symptoms of dyspepsia and nausea, they are not generally recommended for cytoprotective purposes. There is not any better evidence for a cytoprotective effect of sucralfate. In 1989 a prostaglandin analog, misoprostol (Cytotec), was marketed under the sole indication of preventing NSAID-induced mucosal injury. Premarketing studies involving aspirin and other NSAIDs suggested a significant cytoprotective effect and up to a 93% reduction in ulcer development. The recommended dosage is 200 μg qid, but some protection results from lower doses. Side effects are relatively minor and have consisted primarily of diarrhea. Misoprostol has no value in treating or preventing symptoms, and its ulcer-healing effect has not been proven though it is antisecretory. Just when it is indicated is an issue of current debate. The cost alone is sufficient to discourage routine use, and it is usually recommended for patients at high risk for mucosal injury, especially those with previously documented gastric lesions and the elderly.

Several small studies have addressed the healing of gastric, esophageal, and duodenal lesions treated with various ulcer regimens in the face of continued NSAID therapy, and the results have been contradictory. Presently the prudent course would be to avoid any NSAID in a patient known to have an active lesion, and even for several months after healing has been documented. A number of other rather arbitrary recommendations can be made also. Perhaps the most obvious is to avoid regular anti-inflammatory doses of any NSAID unless a definite indication exists. Whenever possible non-acetylated salicylate or enteric-coated aspirin might be used instead of the agents thought to be more strongly associated with mucosal injury. Patients should be warned not just about symptoms but also about the signs of occult blood loss. Some maneuver aimed at detecting chronic occult bleeding, such as periodic hemoglobin determinations, should be planned at the onset of therapy. Special precautions should be employed in patients with a history of gastropathy (or esophageal or duodenal disease) and in the elderly, and prophylactic therapy with misoprostol should be considered in these high-risk subjects. Any evidence for bleeding should result in prompt discontinuation of the NSAID and in a proper investigation.

Lower gastrointestinal tract pathology resulting from NSAIDs is less well defined. Reports have linked NSAIDs with worsening of inflammatory bowel disease symptoms. Diarrhea has been frequently reported and may occur most often with meclofenamate. A few cases of perforated colonic diverticuli have been associated with NSAID use. Constipation is probably the most commonly reported symptom and it may occur more often with the salicylates than with other agents.

The use of enteric-coated aspirin deserves special comment in this section. Dissolution of the coating is pH-dependent; therefore, the tablet passes through the stomach intact if the pH is less than about 4 (variable depending on the preparation). Obstructive bezoars have been reported in patients with pyloric stenosis. Although not yet investigated, it seems likely that pharmacologic or surgical manipulations aimed at raising gastric pH could result in partial or complete intragastric dissolution of the tablet and at least defeat the purpose of the coating; therefore, concomitant use of enteric-coated aspirin and an H_2-blocker is not recommended. Erratic absorption has been a long-standing concern, but most of the agents currently used have not demonstrated this problem when adequately studied; however, it might be wise to avoid the use of generic preparations. It is not entirely clear why enteric coating protects the gastric mucosa, but the effect is likely related to avoiding the sustained toxicity of acetylsalicylic acid trapped in the gastric mucosal cell at its site of absorption.

MISCELLANEOUS REACTIONS

Numerous possible reactions have been reported in small series or as isolated case reports; the most important of these are summarized in Table 2-8. Only the hematologic reactions require comment here. All of the NSAIDs impair platelet aggregation, but, except for aspirin, the effect is reversible within a few half-lives of discontinuing the agent. Clinically significant bleeding episodes have rarely been reported, but patients commonly complain of abnormal bruising. The effect may aggravate upper gastrointestinal bleeding from peptic ulcers or NSAID gastropathy, and it may be important at surgery; therefore, it is usually recommended that these agents be discontinued prior to elective surgery.

Table 2-8. Uncommon miscellaneous NSAID side effects

Side effect	Major agent(s)
Acute pulmonary edema	Salicylates (usually in toxic doses)
Hypersensitivity pneumonitis	Naproxen, ibuprofen, sulindac, phenylbutazone, and others
Stomatitis	Any agent
Sialadenitis	Phenylbutazone and others
Febrile reactions	Ibuprofen
Drug-induced lupus erythematosus	Phenylbutazone, ibuprofen
Carditis	Phenylbutazone
Vasculitis	Phenylbutazone, indomethacin, and naproxen
Pancreatitis	Sulindac and others
Acute proctocolitis	Mefenamic acid, aspirin

A few cases of aplastic anemia have been reported in patients taking aspirin, indomethacin, sulindac, diclofenac, ibuprofen, fenoprofen, naproxen, and piroxicam, but phenylbutazone is the only NSAID regularly reported to cause such a reaction. Its routine association with aplastic anemia may render it too toxic for almost any use. Otherwise isolated reports link various NSAIDs to cases of pure red cell aplasia, thrombocytopenia, neutropenia, and hemolytic anemia. The infrequency of these occurrences does not seem to justify regular complete blood counts for purposes of toxicity monitoring, except when phenylbutazone is used regularly.

DRUG INTERACTIONS

Interactions of other drugs and NSAIDs do not commonly cause clinical problems except perhaps in the elderly and in individuals with renal disease; however, NSAIDs should be avoided whenever possible in patients taking anticoagulants of any type. Potentially important NSAID drug interactions are summarized in Table 2-9.

Relative Expense

A number of variables influence the cost of a regular NSAID program. In addition to the agent prescribed, these include the dose, the availability of generic preparations, the particular facility dispensing the prescription, the month and year the drug is purchased, and whether or not a prescription is required. Among the commonly used salicylates, only aspirin is available in a pure form without prescription, and ibuprofen is the only nonprescription nonsalicylate NSAID available. Other than the salicylates, phenylbutazone, indomethacin, fenoprofen, ibuprofen, sulindac, and meclofenamate are available in generic forms. Most of the nongeneric, nonsalicylate NSAIDs are priced so that a month's supply of a maximum dose will differ little among them. In mid-1991 that price would be in the range of $60/month. The nonacetylated salicylates would be

Table 2-9. Potentially important NSAID drug interactions

Drug	Nature of interaction
Aminoglycosides	Increased aminoglycoside level (related to decreased renal function).
Antacids	NSAID absorption may be reduced by aluminum-containing compounds.
Anticoagulants	May prolong warfarin effect; may increase likelihood of gastrointestinal bleeding.
Barbiturates	May accelerate NSAID metabolism.
Cholestyramine	May inhibit NSAID absorption.
Digoxin	Increased digoxin level (related to decreased renal function).
Hypoglycemic agents	NSAID may potentiate hypoglycemic effect.
Lithium	NSAID may decrease renal excretion.
Phenytoin	NSAID may inhibit phenytoin metabolism.
Potassium-sparing diuretics	Increased likelihood of hyperkalemia with NSAID.
Uricosuric drugs	May reduce renal clearance and metabolism of NSAIDs.
Valproate	NSAID may inhibit valproate metabolism.

somewhat less. Prescription (Zorprin, Easprin) or nonprescription (Ecotrin) aspirin and generic salsalate can be expected to cost about half as much as a nongeneric prescription NSAID. The addition of misoprostol to any NSAID program can be expected to double its cost.

Bibliography

BASIC PHARMACOLOGY

Abramson, S. B., and Weissmann, G. The mechanisms of action of nonsteroidal antiinflammatory drugs. *Arthritis Rheum.* 32:1–9, 1989.

Altman, R. Neutrophil activation: an alternative to prostaglandin inhibition as the mechanism of action for NSAIDs. *Semin. Arthritis Rheum.* 19:1–5, 1990.

Boynton, C. S., Dick, C. F., and Mayor, G. H. NSAIDs: An overview. *J. Clin. Pharmacol.* 28:512–517, 1988.

Day, R. O., et al. Variability in response to NSAIDs: Fact or fiction? *Drugs* 36:643–651, 1988.

Dunn, M. J., et al. Nonsteroidal anti-inflammatory drugs and renal function. *J. Clin. Pharmacol.* 28:524–529, 1988.

Furst, D. E. Clinically important interactions of nonsteroidal anti-inflammatory drugs with other medications. *J. Rheumatol.* 15:58–62, 1988.

Hochberg, M. C. NSAIDs: Mechanisms and pathways of action. *Hosp. Pract.* 24:185–198, 1989.

Lanza, F. L. A review of mucosal protection by synthetic prostaglandin

E analogs against injury by non-steroidal anti-inflammatory agents. *Scand. J. Gastroenterol.* 24:36–43, 1989.

Lin, J. H., Coccheto, D. M., and Duggan, D. E. Protein binding as a primary determinant of the clinical pharmacokinetic properties of nonsteroidal anti-inflammatory drugs. *Clin. Pharmacokinet.* 12:402–432, 1987.

Miners, J. O. Drug interactions involving aspirin (acetylsalicylic acid) and salicylic acid. *Clin. Pharmacokinet.* 17:327–344, 1989.

Netter, P., Bannwarth, B., and Royer-Morrot, M. J. Recent findings on the pharmacokinetics of non-steroidal anti-inflammatory drugs in synovial fluid. *Clin. Pharmacokinet.* 17:145–162, 1989.

Nicosia, S., and Patrono, C. Eicosanoid biosynthesis: Novel opportunities for pharmacological intervention. *FASEB J.* 3:1941–1948, 1989.

Oates, J. A. Antagonism of antihypertensive drug therapy by nonsteroidal anti-inflammatory drugs. *Hypertension* 11:4–6, 1988.

Patrono, C. Aspirin and human platelets: from clinical trials to acetylation of cyclooxygenase and back. *TIPS* 10:453–458, 1989.

Patrono, C. Renal prostaglandins: Biochemistry and functional significance in man. *Contrib. Nephrol.* 69:55–66, 1989.

Simon, L. S., and Mills, J. A. Nonsteroidal antiinflammatory drugs 1,2. *N. Engl. J. Med.* 302:1179–1185, 1237–1243, 1980.

Todd, P. A., and Sorkin, E. M. Diclofenac sodium: A reappraisal of its pharmacodynamic and pharmacokinetic properties, and therapeutic efficacy. *Drugs* 35:244–285, 1988.

CLINICAL INDICATIONS

Abramson, S. B. Therapy and mechanisms of nonsteroidal anti-inflammatory drugs. *Curr. Opinion Rheumatol.* 1:61–67, 1989.

Binus, M. H., Lyon, J. A., and Nicholas, J. L. Comparable serum salicylate concentrations from choline magnesium trisalicylate, aspirin, and buffered aspirin in rheumatoid arthritis. *Arthritis Rheum.* 25:464–466, 1982.

Brooks, P. M., and Day, R. O. Nonsteroidal antiinflammatory drugs—differences and similarities. *N. Engl. J. Med.* 324:1716–1725, 1991.

Cassell, S., et al. Steady-state serum salicylate levels in hospitalized patients with rheumatoid arthritis. *Arthritis Rheum.* 22:384–388, 1979.

Cush, J. J., et al. Relationship between clinical efficacy and laboratory correlates of inflammatory and immunologic activity in rheumatoid arthritis patients treated with nonsteroidal antiinflammatory drugs. *Arthritis Rheum.* 33:623–633, 1990.

Furst, D. E., et al. A controlled study of concurrent therapy with a non-acetylated salicylate and naproxen in rheumatoid arthritis. *Arthritis Rheum.* 30:146–154, 1987.

Furst, D. E., et al. A strategy for reaching therapeutic salicylate levels in patients with rheumatoid arthritis using standardized dosing regimens. *J. Rheumatol.* 14:342–347, 1987.

Kolodny, A. L. Two double blind trials of diclofenac sodium with aspirin and with naproxen in the treatment of patients with rheumatoid arthritis. *J. Rheumatol.* 15:1205–1211, 1988.

Luggen, M. E., Gartside, P. S., and Hess E. V. Nonsteroidal antiinflammatory drugs in rheumatoid arthritis: duration of use as a measure of relative value. *J. Rheumatol.* 16:1565–1569, 1989.

Multicenter Salsalate/Aspirin Comparison Study Group. Does the acetyl group of aspirin contribute to the antiinflammatory efficacy of salicylic acid in the treatment of rheumatoid arthritis? *J. Rheumatol.* 16:321–327, 1989.

Pincus, T., and Callahan, L. F. Clinical use of multiple nonsteroidal antiinflammatory drug preparations within individual rheumatology private practices. *J. Rheumatol.* 16:1253–1258, 1989.

Schlegel, S. I., and Paulus, H. E. Update on NSAID use in rheumatic diseases. *Bull. Rheum. Dis.* 36:1–8, 1986.

SIDE EFFECTS

Barrier, C. H., and Hirschowitz, B. I. Controversies in the detection and management of nonsteroidal anti-inflammatory drug-induced side effects of the upper gastrointestinal tract. *Arthritis Rheum.* 32:926–932, 1989.

Carson, J. L. et al. The relative gastrointestinal toxicity of the nonsteroidal anti-inflammatory drugs. *Arch. Intern. Med.* 147:1054–1057, 1987.

Cryer, B., Goldschmiedt, M., Redfern, J. S., and Feldman, M. Comparison of salsalate and aspirin on mucosal injury and gastroduodenal mucosal prostaglandins. *Gastroenterology* 99:1616–1621, 1990.

Fries, J. F. et al. Toward an epidemiology of gastropathy associated with nonsteroidal antiinflammatory drug use. *Gastroenterology* 96:647–655, 1989.

Graham, D. Y., Agrawal, N. M., and Roth, S. H. Prevention of NSAID-induced gastric ulcer with misoprostol: multicentre, double-blind, placebo-controlled trial. *Lancet* Dec. 3:1277–1280, 1988.

Grigor, R. R., Spitz, P. W., and Furst, D. E. Salicylate toxicity in elderly patients with rheumatoid arthritis. *J. Rheumatol.* 14:60–66, 1987.

Hale, W. E., et al. Renal effects of nonsteroidal anti-inflammatory drugs in the elderly. *Curr. Ther. Res.* 46:173–179, 1989.

Halla, J. T., and Hardin, J. G. Salicylate ototoxicity in patients with rheumatoid arthritis: a controlled study. *Ann. Rheum. Dis.* 47:134–137, 1988.

Hillman, A. L., and Bloom, B. S. Economic effects of prophylactic use of misoprostal to prevent gastric ulcer in patients taking nonsteroidal anti-inflammatory drugs. *Arch. Intern. Med.* 149:2061–2065, 1989.

Lanza, F., et al. An endoscopic comparison of the effects of etodolac, indomethacin, ibuprofen, naproxen, and placebo on the gastrointestinal mucosa. *J. Rheumatol.* 14:338–341, 1987.

Lanza, F., et al. An endoscopic comparison of the gastroduodenal injury seen with salsalate and naproxen. *J. Rheumatol.* 16:1570–1574, 1989.

Lanza, F. L., Royer, G. L., Jr., and Nelson, R. S. Endoscopic evaluation of the effects of aspirin, buffered aspirin, and enteric-coated aspirin on the gastric and duodenal mucosa. *N. Engl. J. Med.* 303:136–138, 1980.

Morassut, P., Yang, W., and Karsh, J. Aspirin intolerance. *Semin. Arthritis Rheum.* 19:22–30, 1989.

O'Brien, W. M., and Bagby, G. F. Rare adverse reactions to nonsteroidal antiinflammatory drugs. *J. Rheumatol.* 12:13–20, 1985.

Petroski, D. Endoscopic comparison of various aspirin preparations—gastric mucosal adaptability to aspirin restudied. *Curr. Ther. Res.* 45:945–954, 1989.

Pullar, T., et al. A study of tolerance to the psychomotor effects of indomethacin in healthy volunteers. *Br. J. Rheumatol.* 28:317–319, 1989.

Roth, S., et al. Reduced risk of NSAID gastropathy (GI mucosal toxicity) with nonacetylated salicylate (salsalate): An endoscopic study. *Semin. Arthritis Rheum.* 19:11–19, 1990.

Simon, L. S. Toxicity of nonsteroidal anti-inflammatory drugs. *Curr. Opinion Rheumatol.* 1:68–73, 1989.

Slepian, I. K., Mathews, K. P., and McLean, J. A. Aspirin-sensitive asthma. *Chest* 87:386–391, 1985.

Soll, A. H., Weinstein, W. M., Kurata, J., and McCarthy, D. Nonsteroidal anti-inflammatory drugs and peptic ulcer disease. *Ann. Intern. Med.* 114:307–319, 1991.

Toto, R. D., et al. Effects of acute and chronic dosing of NSAIDs in patients with renal insufficiency. *Kidney Int.* 30:760–768, 1986.

Waslen, T. A., McCauley, F. A., and Wilson, T. W. Sulindac does not spare renal prostaglandins. *Clin. Invest. Med.* 12:77–81, 1989.

Whelton, A., et al. Renal effects of ibuprofen, piroxicam, and sulindac in patients with asymptomatic renal failure. *Ann. Intern. Med.* 112:568–576, 1990.

Wysenbeek, A. J., et al. Assessment of cognitive function in elderly patients treated with naproxen. A prospective study. *Clin. Exp. Rheumatol.* 6:399–400, 1988.

Corticosteroids

The dramatic effects of cortisone and adrenocorticotropic hormone (ACTH) on the signs and symptoms of active rheumatoid arthritis were first reported by Dr. Hench and his associates in 1949. The consequences of this landmark discovery have affected virtually every area of medicine, especially rheumatology, and the impact has not always been perceived as favorable. For many symptomatic rheumatic diseases, these drugs simply work too well yet have too many side effects.

Whereas all available synthetic corticosteroids will be addressed in the section on basic pharmacology (Table 3-1), the clinical sections will focus on the few that are widely used in rheumatic disease patients. With minor exceptions, the various agents are similar in efficacy and side effects and differ only in potency and duration of action. Perhaps because so few differences exist among the various agents, most rheumatologists habitually use only a limited number, particularly prednisone and methylprednisolone. Because of dosing inconvenience and unpredictable biologic effects, ACTH is rarely used in rheumatic disease practices, though it might be appropriate

Table 3-1. Commonly used available systemic corticosteroid preparations

Name	Preparation(s)	Equivalent potency (mg)
Cortisone acetate	5-mg, 10-mg, 25-mg tablets	25
Hydrocortisone	10-mg, 20-mg tablets; various parenteral preparations (hydrocortisone sodium phosphate 50 mg/ml)	20
Prednisone/ prednisolone	1-mg, 2.5-mg, 5-mg, 10-mg, 20-mg, 50-mg tablets; various parenteral preparations (prednisolone sodium phosphate 20 mg/ml)	5
Methylprednisolone	2-mg, 4-mg, 8-mg, 16-mg, 24-mg, 32-mg tablets; various parenteral preparations (methylprednisolone sodium succinate in varying dilutions)	4
Triamcinolone	1-mg, 2-mg, 4-mg, 8-mg tablets	4
Betamethasone	0.6-mg tablets; various parenteral preparations (betamethasone phosphate 6 mg/ml)	0.75
Dexamethasone	0.25-mg, 0.5-mg, 0.75-mg, 1.5-mg, 6-mg tablets; various parenteral preparations (dexamethasone phosphate 4 mg/ml and 24 mg/ml)	0.75

when a very brief course of therapy is anticipated. A new prednisone derivative, deflazacort, is now under investigation and may be available in this country in the future; it appears to have significantly fewer side effects than currently available agents, and its introduction could be a major advance in corticosteroid therapy. Although many of the principles of corticosteroid therapy addressed in this chapter are applicable to other diseases, only those considered to be rheumatic in nature will be specifically discussed.

Basic Pharmacology

The actions and mechanisms of action of corticosteroids or glucocorticoids, the steroidal anti-inflammatory drugs (SAIDs), are complex; however, some of the anti-inflammatory effects of the SAIDs can be related to the prevention of metabolism of arachidonic acid. In order to use the background already presented concerning arachidonic acid metabolism, this aspect will be covered first. Effects through inhibition of formation of parallel products will be considered also. The means by which liberation of arachidonic acid from membrane phospholipids occurs and is modulated are developed in greater detail in this chapter than in the previous chapter on nonsteroidal anti-inflammatory drugs (NSAIDs): The purpose is to provide a framework for proposed mechanisms of interference with release of arachidonic acid by SAIDs. The reader is referred to Chapter 2 for an overview and also for details of arachidonic acid metabolism subsequent to its liberation.

Significant additional anti-inflammatory effects of the SAIDs can occur through a number of effects on leukocytes, especially neutrophils and monocytes/macrophages. Changes in leukocyte population composition and mediator production are presented, with possible mechanisms. SAIDs influence formation and effects of several inflammation mediators of leukocyte origin, particularly interleukin-1 (IL-1). These effects and some related immunomodulatory effects are reviewed.

Common side effects of SAIDs are only briefly reviewed, as these are generally familiar, and the mechanisms, where known, have changed least in recent time. Basic pharmacologic properties of the SAID class and of some individual members are also presented in this chapter.

STEROID RECEPTORS AND GENERAL
MECHANISMS OF SAID EFFECTS

Endogenous SAIDs (corticosterone/aldosterone, cortisol [hydrocortisone]) are formed from cholesterol by the adrenal cortex under the influence of corticotropin-releasing hormone (hypothalamus) and corticotropin (ACTH; anterior pituitary). ACTH increases the rate-limiting first conversion of cholesterol to pregnenolone, a common precursor for all adrenal steroid end products. Cortisol, the chief SAID, travels via blood to the numerous sites where its effects are exerted. Cortisol in blood is bound to two proteins, one a specific binding protein (corticosteroid-binding globulin [CBG]; transcortin),

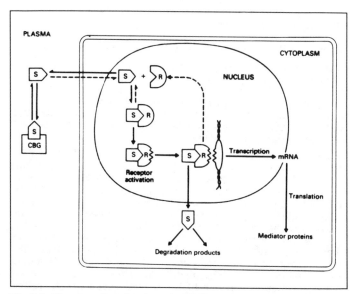

Fig. 3-1. Diagram of mechanism of action of SAIDs on intracellular receptors. (CBG, corticosteroid-binding globulin [in plasma]; S, steroid; R, receptor; mRNA, messenger ribonucleic acid.) (From M. M. Dale and J. C. Foreman (eds.). *Textbook of Immunopharmacology* (2nd ed.). Oxford: Blackwell, 1989. P. 280. With permission.)

the other albumin. The composite extent of binding is about 90%: 80% corticosteroid-binding globulin; 10% albumin.

SAIDs are highly lipophilic and thus readily penetrate cell membranes. Receptors for steroids occur intracellularly, in contrast to the usual surface cell membrane receptors for other hormones, mediators, and so forth. Binding of the steroid to its receptors causes exposure of DNA/chromatin-binding sites on the steroid-receptor complex, followed by translocation of the complex into the cell nucleus, and interaction with specific genes. The result of the latter is activation or inhibition of individual genes, with increases or decreases in expression of, i.e., in the levels of, respective messenger RNA and protein end products. The steps in transport and receptor interaction of steroids are summarized in Fig. 3-1.

Fundamentally, then, all SAID effects can be related to a single effect, i.e., regulation of protein formation, resulting from interaction with specific cytosolic receptors. Complexity immediately enters any consideration of SAID effects, however, because the receptors are widespread and so many different proteins can be influenced. Only a **very** few of the total proteins will be considered here. It is important to note that exogenously administered natural hormone or synthetic analogs act analogously to endogenous hormone, although differences in extent of binding, degree of glucocorticoid versus mineralocorticoid activity, and so forth, occur from one to another.

EFFECTS OF SAID RELATED TO EICOSANOIDS AND PARALLEL PRODUCTS

Additional Mediators Formed by Phospholipase A_2 Action

In chapter 2, on NSAIDs, conversions of arachidonic acid through the cyclooxygenase and lipoxygenase pathways were the main focus. It is appropriate at this point to indicate another possible, and probable, product parallel to arachidonic acid metabolites and initiated by the action of phospholipase A_2 (PLA_2), i.e., platelet-activating factor (PAF). It should be remembered also that arachidonate itself leads to multiple active products.

As was previously mentioned, the usual substrate for PLA_2 is phosphatidylcholine, an abundant phospholipid in cell membranes and one that contains a high percentage of arachidonic acid in the 2-position acted on by the enzyme. An analog of phosphatidyl choline, phosphatid**al** choline, also occurs in membrane lipids, although it occurs to a lesser extent. The only difference between the two lipids occurs in the nature of attachment of the fatty acid to glycerol in the 1-position: In phosphatidyl choline the linkage is an ester bond, whereas in phosphatidal choline the linkage is an ether bond. The ether linkage phospholipids compose the class called **plasmalogens**. Importantly, both phosphatidyl and phosphatidal choline are equally good substrates for PLA_2. Activation of PLA_2, therefore, could liberate arachidonic acid from both lipids.

The lysophospholipid formed from phosphatidyl choline is rapidly remodeled, i.e., the intact phospholipid is regenerated. In contrast, the lysophospholipid from phosphatidal choline can be acetylated in the 2-position to yield sn-2-acetylglycerophosphocholine, or PAF. An overall scheme and reference structures are provided in Fig. 3-2.

Although it is called **platelet**-activating factor, in deference to its ability to cause platelet aggregation and release, PAF has significant effects on other cells. The most abundant producers of PAF include platelets, neutrophils, macrophages (monocytes?), and eosinophils. PAF is chemotactic for neutrophils and elicits neutrophil release, including proteases. It is also a potent vasodilator, elicits direct, long-lasting increases in vascular permeability, and is a potent bronchoconstrictor. Indeed, a role for PAF in the etiology of asthma is becoming widely accepted; however, it is also clear that PAF is a possible mediator of inflammatory reactions.

Highly specific antagonists of PAF at the receptor level are available for research purposes and include some drugs marketed for other purposes (e.g., triazolobenzodiazepines). Specific antagonists of **only** PAF are in various stages of testing. The PAF antagonists are not covered here, as sufficient documentation to indicate any utility in inflammation has not been accomplished. The effects of SAIDs, however, may relate in part to changes in PAF production, elicited through effects on PLA_2.

Regulation of Arachidonic Acid Liberation

As described in chapter 2 on NSAIDs, the rate-limiting step in subsequent conversions of arachidonic acid to its various biologically active end products is availability of free arachidonic acid. The en-

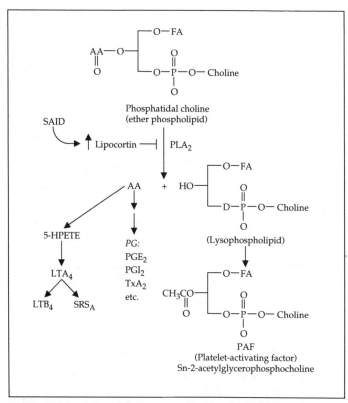

Fig. 3-2. Scheme for parallel generation of platelet-activating factor (PAF) and eicosanoids subsequent to activation of phospholipase A₂ (PLA₂). (—, inhibits; AA, arachidonic acid; FA, fatty acid (usually (C16–C18); HPETE, hydroperoxyeicosatetraenoic acid; LT, leukotriene; PG, prostaglandin; Tx, thromboxane.)

zyme that is responsible for the bulk of arachidonate that is released on stimulation is PLA_2, a membrane-associated enzyme. The activity of PLA_2 is sensitive to intracellular calcium, possibly through a calcium-binding protein. In addition, associated regulatory proteins can affect the activity level of PLA_2.

A main regulatory protein(s) was identified in several tissues by several groups nearly simultaneously, resulting in a number of names, including renocortin, macrocortin, lipomodulin, vasocortin, and endocortin. It is now generally accepted that indeed different proteins exist, ranging in molecular weights from 15,000 to 40,000 (lipomodulin); however, these different proteins are immunologically related and perform a similar function. The lower molecular weight forms may in fact be derived from the 40,000 molecular weight form. In recent history the term **lipocortin** has been adopted for general use (**lipocortins** for the group, **lipocortin** per se for what was previously lipomodulin). Lipocortin has several characteristics that may be involved in its proposed regulatory role for PLA_2.

Lipocortin is highly polar, associates with PLA_2, and, in its native state, acts to inhibit the enzyme. As mentioned in chapter 2 on NSAIDs, many stimuli act through receptors coupled to phospholipase C, the action of which generates (at least) two intracellular messengers, inositol triphosphate (IP_3) and diacylglycerol (DAG). Through its action as a calcium ionophore, IP_3 can mobilize calcium from intracellular storage sites and thus increases free intracellular calcium levels: Calcium-sensitive enzymes such as PLA_2 and 5-lipoxygenase may then be activated. Additional free calcium may be available via entry of extracellular calcium through receptor-operated channels in the plasma membrane. Intracellular phosphorylation reactions can be initiated by DAG stimulation of protein kinase C. One protein that may be phosphorylated is lipocortin, with loss of its PLA_2 inhibitory function. Thus, subsequent to stimulation of a cell and activation of phospholipase C, intracellular calcium increases, and lipocortin is inactivated, allowing for full expression of PLA_2 activity. The inhibitory function of lipocortin can be regenerated by dephosphorylation.

Some controversy exists as to exactly how (and in a few cases, even whether) lipocortin regulates PLA_2. The most common view is that binding of lipocortin to PLA_2 effects a conformational and thus activity change in the enzyme; however, lipocortin can bind calcium and also phospholipids. Based on the latter observation, it has been proposed that lipocortin may bind PLA_2 substrate and prevent its hydrolysis. At present the mechanism(s) of lipocortin is still speculative, although its function is generally accepted, albeit with some reservations.

Many times stimuli are formed or are present only short term and are thus available to cellular receptors only briefly. Based on this simplistic observation, and the mechanisms of stimulus-elicited PLA_2 activation presented so far, it might be expected that changes in PLA_2 activity would be temporally linked to stimulus availability. Indeed, stimulus-elicited formation of arachidonate metabolites is usually observed to be very brief; however, evidence exists to indicate that some stimuli can elicit synthesis of a PLA_2-activating protein (PLAP). The actions of this protein are basically the reverse of lipocortin: The protein binds to PLA_2 and activates it or it binds substrate and enhances its utilization, or a combination of these. Whether increases in PLAP contribute to increased basal or elicited formation of inflammatory arachidonate products, or both, or to longer-term changes as a result of finite stimulation, is not known currently.

SAID Regulation of Lipocortin Levels

Once the mechanism of action of the NSAIDs, i.e., limitation of prostanoid formation via inhibition of cyclooxygenase, was realized, similar actions were investigated for the SAIDs. It was quickly realized that the SAIDs had no ability to directly interact with cyclooxygenase, i.e., with the metabolism of arachidonic acid per se; however, it was subsequently documented that stimulated formation of arachidonic acid metabolites was in fact decreased by SAIDs.

Because levels of free arachidonic acid are extremely low, SAID-decreased release of arachidonic acid was identified as the probable mechanism. Knowledge of the abundance and position of arachidonic acid in membrane phospholipids, and of the enzymes that could hydrolyze it from substrate, indicated PLA_2 action as the probable means of liberation. These observations provided the foundation for further delineation of the mechanism of steroid anti-inflammatory effects.

Additional observations relative to SAID action are important in defining their mechanism. The first observation was that a significant time lag (minutes to many hours in some tissues) occurred after addition of the steroid until an effect could be demonstrated. Another was that SAIDs were completely without effect in cell-free homogenates. Inhibitors of various steps involved in protein synthesis initiated at the level of the nucleus were found to prevent steroid-induced decreases in arachidonate availability/end product formation. Subsequently, the various peptides that compose the lipocortins were isolated and characterized, and dose-response relationships between the level of steroid and level of lipocortin were documented. Importantly, levels of natural steroid that are commonly in the circulation fall within the anti-inflammatory dose-response range, indicating steroid regulation of PLA_2, through lipocortin, to be a probable physiologic phenomenon. That anti-inflammatory effects are physiologically regulated by steroids is supported by the intense inflammatory and hyperalgesic responses that result from adrenalectomy.

Presently, not only has lipocortin itself been purified and sequenced, its gene has been isolated and cloned. Steroid treatment of cells can be shown to increase the mRNA for lipocortin, thus providing direct data to support the indirect data from RNA or protein synthesis inhibition or both by various drugs (e.g., actinomycin D, puromycin, cycloheximide).

A defect in natural SAID (cortisol) regulation of PLA_2 in chronic, severe inflammatory states has been suggested. The origin of the suggestion is the observation that a high percentage of people with inflammatory disorders have circulating levels of autoantibodies to lipocortin. This observation is in keeping with the long-standing suggestion that rheumatoid arthritis and other disease states characterized by widespread inflammatory responses have an auto-immune basis. Clearly additional systems are involved, as other autoantibodies are frequently seen, including rheumatoid factor (anti-immunoglobulin G [IgG]) and collagen antibodies. The latter are generally observed after some progression of the disease and have been suggested to be elicited by ongoing damage. It is intriguing, although undocumented, to speculate an early involvement of deregulation of a natural anti-inflammatory system. If indeed such a defect is an early and major factor in evolution of the disease, therapy aimed at restoring lipocortin function might be very beneficial.

Lipocortin itself has been used experimentally to effect anti-inflammatory activity. The effects are significant and can be achieved by systemic or more restricted administration. Use of a relatively large protein such as lipocortin as a drug is possible, but this poses a number of problems, including that oral administration is precluded. Also, as a protein, an immune reaction to it might occur, and, in circumstances where auto-antibodies already exist, the immune reaction to it could be enhanced; however, an understanding of lipocortin's exact mechanism(s) of interaction with, and effect on, PLA_2 could lead to development of new drugs that could bypass the well-known side effects of steroid administration. Several proteins with similar actions to lipocortin and also lipid inhibitors of PLA_2 are under investigation.

Consequences of PLA₂ Inhibition

Since the liberation of arachidonic acid is rate-limiting for the production of end products of **both** pathways of arachidonate metabolism, SAID inhibition of PLA_2 translates to decreases in prostanoids, hydroperoxy derivatives, and also leukotrienes. A broad spectrum of potential participants in inflammation is thus reduced.

Several side effects of SAIDs are similar to some for the NSAIDs. For example, some evidence shows increased risk of peptic ulceration. The latter is clearly not of the magnitude of occurrence initially suspected, although lesions can progress "silently" and thus not present until in a severe stage because of the potent anti-inflammatory, and thus pain-limiting, properties of the SAIDs. The mechanisms of lesion occurrence can still be related in part to decreased gastric production of protective prostanoids (PGE_2, PGI_2). As mentioned in chapter 2, on NSAIDs, some evidence exists that gastric (gastrointestinal) side effects relate not simply to decreased prostanoid production, but to an imbalance in the production of lipoxygenase metabolites versus cyclooxygenase metabolites, an imbalance that shunting of substrate could intensify. The less than anticipated occurrence of gastric problems could perhaps reflect inhibition of **both** pathways by SAIDs, keeping the balance intact.

Renal side effects of the NSAID type related to decreased renal vascular prostanoid production do not seem to occur with steroids; however, steroid use may result in an elevation of blood pressure in some individuals, and this has been suggested to result from impairment of vascular prostacyclin production. The hypertensive changes due to decreased prostacyclin could be partially offset by other effects of the steroids (e.g., increased numbers of vasodilator $beta_2$-adrenergic receptors).

OTHER ANTI-INFLAMMATORY EFFECTS OF SAIDs

Altered Leukocyte Populations and Activation

Chronic inflammation sites are characterized by the presence of large quantities of two types of cells in particular, i.e., neutrophils and monocytes/macrophages. Neutrophils arrive early at sites of inflammation and may initiate vascular permeability changes; neutrophil presence is sustained throughout acute and chronic phases of inflammation. Monocyte infiltration begins later and is likewise sustained. These two cell types probably account for a major portion of inflammatory mediators, such as leukotriene B_4 (LTB_4) and IL-1, that are found at the sites.

Several actions of SAIDs on populations and behavior of peripheral leukocytes may be involved in their anti-inflammatory actions. An early action of SAIDs is a reduction in circulating numbers of lymphocytes, eosinophils, basophils, and particularly monocytes, accompanied by an increase in neutrophils. The responsiveness of leukocytes, extending to most populations, is also reduced. This reduction may relate in part to membrane stabilization, extending even to lysosomal stabilization.

The composition of the peripheral leukocyte population is determined by both redistribution and activity changes. For example, the early increase in neutrophils that is observed may reflect increased release from bone marrow as well as decreased exit from the circulation to sites of inflammation. A sustained increase in neutrophils is also common and may result primarily from reduced circulatory egress. Neutrophils may be rendered less responsive broad spectrum, which is a main cause of their decreased exodus from blood, by alterations in intracellular cyclic AMP (cAMP) or changes in surface receptors, or both, as well as by SAID-induced decreases in chemoattractants.

Reductions in non-neutrophil leukocyte populations appear to result primarily from redistribution phenomena. Lymphocytes consist of two main types: T-, or thymus processed, cells and B-, or bone marrow (only) processed, cells. Many B cells are short-lived and stationary, whereas many T cells are longer-lived and migratory, i.e., they circulate from the blood, through high endothelial venules, into lymphoid tissues (lymph nodes, spleen, bone marrow) and enter blood again. Decreases in lymphocytes effected by steroids reflect mainly movement of T-lymphocytes into lymphoid tissues. The mechanism(s) by which this redistribution occurs is speculative and could involve changes in (relative balance of) surface receptors or cAMP levels, or both, as for neutrophils. On long-term administration, decreases in lymphoid tissue mass may also occur, probably due to overall catabolic effects of the SAIDs.

Some of the more outstanding decreases in leukocyte populations involve eosinophils and monocytes. Decreases in the former may have special significance for allergy responses, whereas decreases in the latter would render them less available and thus decrease their participation at sites of inflammation. Since monocytes are also the source of tissue macrophages, populations and contributions of macrophages also may be reduced. In addition to simply making the cells less available, activation of monocytes and macrophages is reduced by steroids. The mechanisms may be similar to those for neutrophils, although SAIDs additionally reduce receptors for IgG (F_c portion) and for complement (C_{3b}) on these cells. Intercellular signals released by monocytes/macrophages are also decreased by SAIDs, with significant impact on the inflammatory cascade.

Cytokines and SAIDs

A comprehensive review of nonprostanoid leukocyte mediators that may be involved in inflammation is outside the scope of this handbook; however, in order to understand the effects of SAIDs that may be related to their influence on these mediators, a basic groundwork is desirable and follows.

The term **cytokines** is used to describe a large group of compounds, mostly small proteins, that regulate both the appearance and the activation of various leukocytes involved in inflammation as well as the proliferation of leukocytes involved in immune responses. One group of cytokines compose the interleukins, a group in which there currently may be more than 12 different members. IL-1 is a cytokine that derives from monocytes/macrophages (and is therefore a monokine, as is a parallel monocytic cytokine, tumor necrosis factor [TNF$_\alpha$], which may also have a role in some inflammatory reactions). Elaboration of IL-1 by monocytic leukocytes is intimately involved in establishing and maintaining an inflammatory "cascade" (see Mechanisms of Metabolic Side Effects of SAIDs).

Resting monocytes have no mRNA for IL-1, but levels rise rapidly subsequent to stimulus exposure. Stimuli can include LTB$_4$, immune complexes, complement (5a), thrombin, and also other cytokines, e.g., lymphokines, a group of cytokines produced by lymphocytes, from lymphocytes activated by antigen or other stimuli. The lymphokines include macrophage-activating factor (MAF; priming signal for subsequent stimulus activation), migration inhibitory factor (MIF; decreased migration can be, confusingly, a sign of activation), and also IL-2. Although IL-1 is the major focus of much of the rest of this chapter, it is important to note that lymphokines can also contribute to inflammation through the following effects: increased neutrophil adherence, aggregation, phagocytosis; chemotaxis of neutrophils, eosinophils, and basophils; osteoclast activation and bone resorption, independent of PGE$_2$ formation; some ability to increase capillary permeability; and stimulation of granulocyte formation/release from bone marrow.

It should be noted that two forms of IL-1 exist, under control of two separate genes: IL-1$_\alpha$ and IL-1$_\beta$. The receptors acted on, and biologic activity of, both forms are very similar. Because of the similar activity, and also since in most cases both forms are affected, the effects of the SAIDs on IL-1 will be referred simply to IL-1, without distinction to subforms. In a few instances, only one form is (currently) documented to be affected, and this will be indicated.

The effects of IL-1 are numerous. IL-1 is identical with endogenous pyrogen, and thus elevation of body temperature is probably its best-known effect. Other effects of IL-1 include elicitation of eicosanoid release (neutrophils, fibroblasts, endothelial cells, synovial cells); hyperalgesia (possibly related to eicosanoid release); secretion of metalloproteinase (chondrocytes) and collagenase (fibroblasts, synovial cells, osteoclasts), thus promoting cartilage/collagen degradation; increased adhesion of neutrophils, monocytes, and lymphocytes; neutrophil and lymphocyte chemotaxis; neutrophil activation; cellular proliferation (fibroblasts, synovial cells, endothelial cells); accelerated procoagulant/decreased plasminogen activator production, and synthesis/exposure of (additional) adhesion molecules by endothelium; angiogenesis; and formation of other IL.

The additional IL elicited by IL-1 include IL-2, a T cell product (lymphokine) that can in turn enhance clonal expansion and function of other lymphocyte populations; IL-4 and IL-5, which stimulate T-helper cells (T_{h2} subset) and IL-6 (also known as interferon β_2), which is involved in immunoglobulin production (differentiation) by B cells and possibly in hepatic production of acute-phase proteins.

In addition to the impressively long list already given, IL-1 may be involved in the well-known hematologic changes characteristic of chronic inflammatory states: Anemia may occur through IL-1 antagonism of the effects of erythropoietin, whereas increases in circulating neutrophils and monocytes may be favored by IL-1–elicited increases in production and effect of colony-stimulating factors (G-CSF, GM-CSF). The effects of the other monokine, TNF_α, include stimulation of PGE_2 formation and collagenase release by synovial cells and could thus amplify the effects of IL-1 as well.

With the list of effects in hand, it is almost anticlimactic to state that SAIDs limit the formation of IL-1, and through this one main effect additionally limit the levels and thus effects of other cytokines. Increases in IL-1 mRNA subsequent to cell stimulation are prevented. There is also some evidence that IL-1$_\beta$ mRNA is destabilized, i.e., its residence time in cells is decreased. The effects of preformed IL-1 may also be limited by SAIDs: IL-1 treatment does not elicit IL-4, IL-5, IL-6, t-PA, or collagenase expression in SAID-treated systems, and, due to SAID effects on PLA_2, eicosanoid formation is also prevented. Granulopoiesis is suppressed by SAIDs, and, characteristically, hematocrit is increased. In summary, anti-inflammatory, immunomodulatory, and hematologic effects of SAIDs can be rationally related to the SAIDs' ability to decrease IL-1 production and effects. The positive feedback, or amplification, relationships that can occur between eicosanoid effects and IL-1 (direct and dependent) effects are also disrupted by SAIDs.

One last relationship between IL-1 and cortisol should be noted, namely the ability of IL-1 to elicit increases in cortisol. Increased cortisol is postulated to be part of a negative feedback loop limiting both the production and effects of IL-1. Limitation of IL-1 effects may actually be promoted by a synergy of IL-6 and cortisol (SAIDs) on release of acute-phase proteins (including antiproteases).

MECHANISMS OF METABOLIC SIDE EFFECTS OF SAIDs

As with the wanted effects of SAIDs, the unwanted effects, mostly on metabolism, relate directly or indirectly to changes in expression of various proteins. Complete separation of SAID effects on metabolism from anti-inflammatory effects by structural modification has **not** been possible, although considerable separation has been achieved (Table 3-2). Despite the latter, any systemic use, or even systemic access, of SAIDs for any extended period is likely to produce some degree of metabolic derangement. The immunomodulatory effects, some of which may be desired, also can be problematic in the face of continuous exposure of treated individuals to infection and thus the need to mount effective immune responses. Immunomodulatory effects could also compromise immune surveillance. Since cortisol modulates its own production (CRH-ACTH levels are inversely related to cortisol levels), high levels of SAIDs for prolonged periods can suppress production of CRH and thus production of ACTH; prolonged lack of ACTH can in turn result in adrenal atro-

Table 3-2. General classification of SAIDs

Steroid	Carbohydrate potency* (mg)	Anti-inflammatory potency	Sodium-retaining potency	Biologic half-life (hr)
Cortisol	20	1	1	8–12
Prednisolone (Δ¹-cortisone)	5	4	0.5	12–36
6-α-Methylprednisolone	4	5	0.5	12–36
9-α-Fluorocortisol	0.1	10	125	12–36
Triamcinolone (9-α-fluoro-16-hydroxyprednisolone)	4	5	0.1	12–36
Betamethasone (9-α-16-β-methylprednisolone)	0.6	25	0.05	36–54
Dexamethasone (9-α-fluoro-16-α-methylprednisolone)	1	30	0.05	36–54

*Carbohydrate action of SAIDs is defined as the stimulation of glucose formation, diminution of its utilization, and promotion of its storage as glycogen.
Source: C. R. Craig and R. E. Stitzel (eds.). *Modern Pharmacology* (2nd ed.). Boston: Little, Brown, 1986. P. 877. With permission.

phy. The metabolic effects of SAIDs are briefly covered here. In reviewing the metabolic effects of SAIDs, it may be of interest to keep in mind that these could be enhanced by (high levels of) one of the cytokines (monokines) mentioned earlier, i.e., TNF_α, which can be formed in parallel with IL-1. The original name of TNF_α was **cachexin**, in deference to its pronounced metabolic effects.

The overall effects of cortisol and the SAIDs on carbohydrate metabolism are diabetogenic, although whether significant increases in blood glucose will be observed in a particular individual cannot be predicted easily. Increased blood glucose is made likely by several different SAID-initiated changes, involving not only carbohydrate metabolism directly, but also indirectly via changes in protein and lipid metabolism.

Catabolism of protein, which results in characteristic decreases in muscle mass, increases availability of amino acids for gluconeogenesis: Liver transamination reactions generate excess glucose, which may increase liver glycogen stores and elevate blood glucose. Other effects of SAIDs may also contribute to increased glucose, e.g., increases in (liver) glucose 6-phosphatase and some transaminases. Insulin receptor synthesis/expression can be increased by SAIDs, which might tend to offset some of the other blood glucose–increasing effects.

Lipolysis is increased by SAIDs, although not to the same extent in all adipose. Lipolysis increases free fatty acid levels and makes glycerol available. The former predisposes to ketosis whereas the latter can contribute to elevations in glucose (glycerol can be converted to glucose in a reversal of glycolysis initiated by glycerokinase).

Although many SAIDs currently in use have minimal mineralocorticoid activity, cortisol and some SAIDs have measurable mineralocorticoid effects. Aldosterone, the main endogenous mineralocorticoid, increases the number or function, or both, of $Na^+ - K^+$ exchange proteins in distal nephron segments. The consequences of enhanced aldosterone-like activity are increased absorption of Na^+ (and thus Cl^- and water) coupled to increased excretion of K^+. The resulting increased volume load may contribute to blood pressure elevation, whereas K^+ losses may contribute to symptoms (weakness) resulting from catabolism-induced decreases in muscle mass.

The list of SAID effects is long enough to be boggling. In this section on unwanted effects of SAIDs, one last example of an effect via protein expression regulation will be mentioned. Thinning of skin induced by SAIDs may be related to decreased synthesis of skin collagen precursor.

Special Features of Specific SAIDs

The structures of cortisone and hydrocortisone (cortisol) are shown in Fig. 3-3; the rings are labeled alphabetically, and positions that undergo modification in the various rings to produce commonly used SAIDs are also indicated. Actual substitutions occurring in the most commonly used SAIDs are listed beneath the structures for reference.

Successful structural modifications of native hormone (cortisol) and precursor (cortisone) to increase anti-inflammatory potency and duration of action are exemplified by the analogs included in Fig. 3-3. Inclusion of a double bond in ring A, position 1,2, or addition of a fluorine in ring C, position 9, increases potency and decreases biotransformation/increases duration of action. Additional increases in potency are effected by ring D, position 16 substitutions, particularly by methylation. Although all SAIDs bind to CBG to some extent, the 16-methyl derivatives are considerably less bound, which probably enhances their overall potency by increasing the free (active) fraction of drug per dose. Potency comparisons of the SAIDs for major pharmacologic effects, and also for duration of effect, are given in Table 3-2.

SAIDs undergo hepatic metabolism, generally a reduction of the ring A, position 11-keto group, followed by conjugation through the resulting 11-hydroxyl group. Although generally the SAIDs do not contribute to drug interactions through protein binding, there is some suggestion that long-term administration may induce hepatic enzymes, including those that convert salicylates. Concomitant administration of SAIDs and a salicylate has been suggested to increase salicylate elimination, but this is not well documented. The potential for interactions via biotransformation reactions should be kept in mind for salicylates as well as other drugs.

Clinical Indications

The clinical indications for SAID therapy in patients with rheumatic diseases will be discussed in two sections: indications for the use of

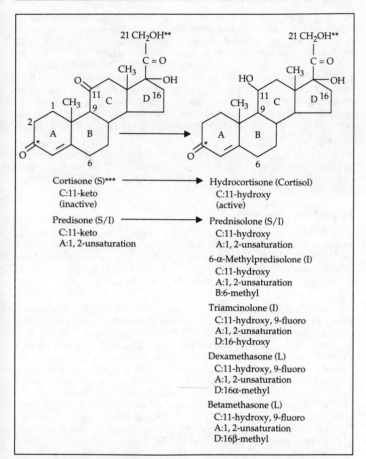

Fig. 3-3. Structures of major commonly used oral/injectable SAIDs. (*, most common site of biotransformation [reduction → conjugation, liver]; **, esterification yields water-soluble form; ***, duration of action [S, short, I, intermediate, L, long].)

the insoluble or depot preparations and the indications for systemic therapy. Unwanted effects of intralesional therapy will be addressed along with its indications, since side effects not only influence the choice of preparation but also dictate its pattern of usage; furthermore, the systemic effects of the depot preparations are minimal, so their side effects differ from those of the systemic preparations.

INSOLUBLE SAIDs

The most widely used depot SAID preparations available in this country are listed in Table 3-3. All can be used for intra-articular or other intralesional (e.g., tendon, bursa, enthesis) injections. Without local anesthesia the injections are painful, and intra-articular

Table 3-3. Available depot SAID preparations

Trade/generic name	Formulation	Disadvantages/advantages
Hydrocortone acetate/ hydrocortisone acetate	25 mg/ml suspension	Less potent than others; can be mixed with local anesthetic
Hydeltra-T.B.A./ prednisolone terbutate	20 mg/ml suspension	Skin atrophy uncommon; can be mixed with local anesthetic
Depo-Medrol/ methylprednisolone acetate	20 mg/ml 40 mg/ml 80 mg/ml suspension	Cannot be mixed with local anesthetic
Aristospan/ triamcinolone hexacetonide	20 mg/ml suspension	May cause more skin atrophy than others; can be mixed with local anesthetic; may be more potent than others
Decadron-LA/ dexamethasone acetate	8 mg/ml suspension	May have more systemic effects than others
Celestone Soluspan/ betamethasone sodium phosphate and betamethasone acetate	3 mg/ml suspension of betamethasone sodium phosphate and 3 mg/ml of betamethasone acetate	Half dose designed for systemic absorption; may be mixed with local anesthetic

injections may rarely result in an acute crystalline-induced synovitis. Pain can be minimized by mixing the SAID with a local anesthetic (when permissible), and the acute synovitis may be preventable by adding a small amount of soluble SAID (such as 0.1 ml of dexamethasone phosphate) to the mixture. Soluble SAID has already been added to the Celestone Soluspan suspension, though it is probably in excess of that needed to prevent the acute reaction. The soluble portion of the mixture will be rapidly absorbed and may result in transient systemic effects, especially if several lesions are injected simultaneously; however, these effects rarely result in clinically apparent SAID toxicity.

The major unwanted effects of intralesional SAID injections of any type are skin atrophy and depigmentation at the site of the injection where a portion of the mixture leaks out into the skin. The leakage is usually unavoidable, but this reaction may be minimized by avoiding the more potent fluorinated preparations such as triamcinolone hexacetonide and betamethasone acetate. More serious concerns with these injections relate to possible joint and tendon damage. Intra-articular injections interfere with chondrocyte metabolism and may accelerate cartilage degeneration as well as weakening joint-supporting structures. Consequently it is recommended that the number of injections per joint be strictly limited, though there is no general agreement as to how limited. For a large weight-bearing joint, once or twice a year might be a reasonable limit. Usually repeated injections become progressively less beneficial in any event. It has been suggested that resting the joint for a few days after the injection might minimize damage (and enhance response), but the value of this maneuver has not been documented. Injections directly into tendons should be avoided (and are difficult to accomplish), but the consequences of injections around tendons and into their sheaths have not been well studied. Achilles tendon rupture has been associated with local SAID injections, but other tendon ruptures have not been clearly related to this practice. Again infrequent injections into the same site can be recommended. Infection has rarely been reported to result from intra-articular or any intralesional injection, though it has been suggested that olecranon bursal injection may predispose to infection at that site. Calcifications have been noted around small hand joints injected with triamcinolone hexacetonide, but these are of doubtful significance.

Advantages and disadvantages of the various insoluble preparations are summarized in Table 3-3. Though it may be less effective than other preparations, prednisolone terbutate has the advantage of causing less skin atrophy and miscibility with a local anesthetic, and will be used here as an example. For an intra-articular injection, one formula might be as follows: 1 part of prednisolone terbutate, one part of 2% lidocaine (perhaps 1.5–2.0 ml each), and a very small amount (perhaps 0.1 ml) of soluble dexamethasone. The dexamethasone can be omitted for extra-articular injections. The amount of total injectant used depends on the size of the joint or other structure targeted. For a large joint such as the hip, knee, or ankle, a total volume of 3–5 ml might be used. For a small hand joint, less than 1 ml will be required. For most bursae and tendons, 3–5 ml can be used. It is generally recommended that all accessible joint and bursal fluid be removed before the injection so as to concentrate the active drug at its site of action. It is also recommended that a force of injection sufficient to rupture the joint capsule not be used.

Common indications for local insoluble SAID injections are summarized in Table 3-4. In patients with rheumatoid arthritis and other chronic inflammatory arthropathies, bursae and tendon sheaths may also be inflamed. Probably the most common indication for depot SAID injections in these patients is persisting inflammation at one or a limited number of sites when the disease is otherwise under adequate control. In this situation a local approach might be preferable to changing or escalating systemic therapy. The possibility of joint infection must always be kept in mind, however; especially in rheumatoid arthritis a major flare in a limited number of joints might represent an infectious episode rather than disease exacerbation. Progressive loss of function of a limited number of joints is another common indication for local therapy. In this situation it might be wise to obtain x-ray films before injecting; a severely damaged joint will not respond to local SAIDs. Whatever the indication for local injection might be, clinically apparent inflammation is a prerequisite. Only inflamed structures can be expected to respond to SAIDs. Because of its limited applicability, local injection should rarely be the mainstay of therapy in patients with systemic rheumatic diseases.

Table 3-4. Common indications for local insoluble SAID injections

Rheumatoid arthritis and other chronic inflammatory arthropathies

    Persisting hand flexor or extensor tenosynovitis—into tendon sheath

    Carpal tunnel syndrome—into tendon sheath or wrist joint

    Elbow flexion contracture with active synovitis—into elbow joint

    Progressive restriction of shoulder range of motion—into shoulder joint

    Baker's cyst—into the knee joint

    Disease flare limited to one or a few sites (exclude infection)—into the inflamed site

Extra-articular or local rheumatic syndromes

    Thumb abductor-extensor tenosynovitis—into the tendon sheaths

    Trigger finger with palpable nodule in volar tendon sheath—into the nodule

    Tennis elbow—into the elbow lateral epicondyle muscle insertion site

    Shoulder rotator cuff tendinitis—over the tender part of the rotator cuff tendon

    Bicipital tenosynovitis—into the tendon sheath of the long head of the biceps

    Trochanteric bursitis—into the tender part of the trochanteric bursa (long needle may be required)

    Anserine bursitis—into the tender part of the anserine bursa

In patients with local rheumatic syndromes, usually tendinitis, bursitis, or enthesopathy, a local injection may be the mainstay of therapy. The alternative is usually days to weeks of a NSAID. As a general rule, the earlier the syndrome is treated, the better the response will be. Controlled studies in this area are rare, but rotator cuff tendinitis has been shown to benefit as well from a single SAID injection as from several days of indomethacin. These data can be used to argue either viewpoint, but the local injection probably has fewer side effects. For most local syndromes incompletely responsive to a single injection, it is probably safe (and often effective) to re-inject once or twice after 7–10 days. It is wise to restrict use of the affected part while determining the effectiveness of the injection. The use of local injections of any type to permit immediate participation in vigorous sporting activities is a practice of doubtful wisdom.

Intra-articular SAID injections are widely used for painful osteoarthritic joints, but this practice is also of doubtful wisdom. Although it is clear that joint inflammation plays some role in the symptoms of osteoarthritis, it is also clear that local steroid injections can accelerate cartilage degeneration. Furthermore, controlled studies have failed to show lasting benefits of knee joint injections in patients with this problem, but data are not available for other joints. Intra-articular depot SAIDs should be used with reluctance, or not at all, in patients with noninflammatory joint disorders.

Few controlled studies of the benefits of local insoluble SAIDs exist in any condition, so it is difficult to define the expectations from such therapy. Obviously this approach seems to work better in patients with self-limiting conditions such as most of the local rheumatic syndromes, since the inflammatory reaction was destined to subside in any event. In patients with chronic arthritis, bursitis, or tenosynovitis, the benefits of a single injection probably last for only a few weeks—12 at most—though that may be long enough for systemic therapy or time enough to bring about a more lasting improvement. Some patients, and perhaps some diseases, may respond better to local depot SAIDs than do others. When considering this approach to therapy, the history of a previous response could be helpful. In systemic diseases this is an adjunctive therapy and usually a temporary one; it should be used with that in mind.

SYSTEMIC SAID THERAPY

Available systemic SAID preparations are summarized in Table 3-1, but this discussion will address only prednisone (or parenteral methylprednisolone) since it is the most widely used synthetic SAID. The reasons for its widespread use are not entirely logical or scientific, but it does have a short-lasting biologic effect that may minimize side effects when large doses are used, and it is available in a number of tablet sizes, which makes it convenient to use. In rheumatology it is seldom possible to generalize concerning systemic SAID use, since dosage schedules, indications, and expectations depend entirely on the disease and its manifestation being treated; however, two generalizations do deserve emphasis: Predictable toxic effects severely limit the use of these agents, and it cannot be proven that they actually favorably alter the outcome of any disease in which they are used. It can be argued that the latter generalization is the result of inadequate data since controlled studies of SAIDs in any rheumatic disease are rare, and it may be—in this case—that absence of proof is not proof of absence. Very judicious use seems indicated, however.

Commonly accepted indications for systemic SAID therapy in the rheumatic diseases are summarized in Table 3-5. Widely variable doses tend to reflect the seriousness or magnitude of the manifestation being treated. Additional less common indications for systemic SAID therapy include the spondyloarthropathies, especially when NSAIDs are contraindicated; polychondritis; acute rheumatic fever; sarcoid arthritis; erythema nodosum; Behçet's syndrome; and the arthritis of inflammatory bowel disease. Initial daily prednisone doses tend to fall into two categories: low (≤ 15 mg) and high (around 60 mg). As a general rule, the low doses are used to treat symptoms and the high doses are used to treat serious or life- or organ-threatening manifestations. Each of these two patterns of use will be discussed separately.

Low-Dose SAIDs

Rheumatoid arthritis is quite literally the prototypical indication for low-dose systemic SAID therapy, but other indications include the less serious manifestations of systemic lupus erythematosus and other connective tissue diseases, some hypersensitivity vasculitis syndromes, and polymyalgia rheumatica. This discussion will focus on rheumatoid arthritis as the example; the same principles can be applied to other indications.

One of the few prospective controlled studies of systemic SAID therapy in any rheumatic disease was published in the mid-1950s. In

Table 3-5. Common indications for systemic SAID therapy in rheumatic disease patients

Disease	Indications	Usual initial daily prednisone dose (mg)
Rheumatoid arthritis	Very active disease unresponsive to NSAIDs	<15
	Necrotizing vasculitis	60
	Pleuritis/pericarditis	15–60
Systemic lupus erythematosus (or mixed connective tissue disease)	Arthritis or minor systemic symptoms unresponsive to NSAIDs	<15
	Nephritis	60
	Serious CNS disease	60
	Thrombocytopenia/hemolytic anemia	30–60
	Systemic vasculitis	30–60
	Pleuritis/pericarditis	15–60
	Myocarditis	60
Poly/dermatomyositis	Inflammatory muscle disease	60
Scleroderma syndromes	Inflammatory muscle disease	30–60
Sjögren's syndrome	Systemic vasculitis	15–60
Systemic-onset juvenile rheumatoid arthritis	Systemic illness including fever unresponsive to NSAIDs	30–60
Systemic necrotizing vasculitis syndromes	Giant-cell arteritis	60
	Polyarteritis nodosa	60
	Wegener's granulomatosis	60
	Most hypersensitivity vasculitis with nephritis	60
	Limited or cutaneous hypersensitivity vasculitis	15–30
Polymyalgia rheumatica	Symptoms	15
Acute crystalline arthritis	Contraindications to use of NSAIDs and colchicine	30
Reflex sympathetic dystrophy	May be an initial therapy	60

that study no advantage of SAIDs over aspirin could be demonstrated over a three-year period in patients with active rheumatoid arthritis. That study and other data accumulated since then have suggested that SAID therapy does not favorably affect long-term outcome in patients with the disease and may predispose to certain deformities. Considering the side effects of these agents, these suggestions serve to severely restrict their indications. Nonetheless the SAIDs are the most rapidly acting and predictably effective anti-inflammatory drugs available, and they will work when the NSAIDs do not; consequently, it is difficult not to use them, but certain empirical rules should be followed.

This therapy should be offered only to patients with clinically apparent active disease unresponsive to nonsteroidal drugs (or when these agents are contraindicated). There should be some plan (such as institution of slow-acting drug therapy) aimed at allowing gradual withdrawal of the SAID at some time in the future. Since symptoms, and not life-threatening manifestations, are being treated, the lowest effective dose should be used. With this in mind, 5 mg/day of prednisone could be started and the dose gradually increased until symptoms were suppressed; more than 10 mg/day is seldom necessary. Since the biologic effects of prednisone are short-lived, the daily requirement should be divided into as many doses as necessary to provide 24-hour comfort; often doses every 8–12 hours are required. Every-other-day schedules are seldom satisfactory, and if they seem to be, immediate withdrawal might be possible.

Perhaps the most important rule concerns gradual withdrawal, not because of adrenal insufficiency concerns, but because of the risk of causing a flare in the disease. Once the patient has shown significant improvement and is relatively comfortable, withdrawal may be begun. The ultimate goal is complete withdrawal, but this practice also permits discovering the lowest dose necessary to sustain comfort. Various schemes have been suggested, but they usually involve decreasing the daily dose by 1 mg every two to four weeks. If worsening results, the previous dose can be resumed and the withdrawal effort repeated in two weeks. An example of the use of systemic SAIDs in active rheumatoid arthritis is illustrated in Fig. 3-4. Unfortunately not all attempted withdrawals will be successful because of failure to otherwise control the disease process, but most probably will. Unless contraindicated, NSAIDs should be continued until corticosteroids are completely withdrawn and no symptoms require therapy.

Sustained-release parenteral SAIDs are sometimes used in patients with rheumatoid arthritis. Examples of these preparations include Decadron-LA and Kenalog-40. These preparations usually allow for a sustained biologic effect equivalent to daily low-dose prednisone over a period of one to three weeks. If these injections are required frequently, low-dose oral prednisone might as well be used. Otherwise these parenteral preparations might be used occasionally to tide a stable patient over a stressful situation when a flare in disease activity is anticipated; however, their effects are not as predictable as those resulting from oral prednisone.

High-Dose SAIDs

Although high-dose SAID therapy is usually regarded as about 60 mg/day of prednisone, much larger doses have been used in a few special situations. No controlled studies define high-dosage schedules or the indications for their use. Consequently the following discussion is based on empiricism and prevailing practice. When used in large doses, the SAIDs are both anti-inflammatory and immunosuppressive; most rheumatic disease clinical situations thought to require these doses could benefit from both actions. No effort will be made to distinguish between them. Many of the sit-

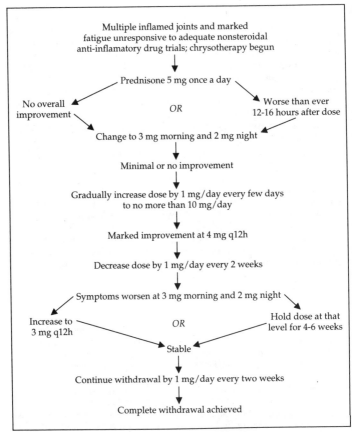

Fig. 3-4. **Example of the use of systemic SAIDs for active rheumatoid arthritis.**

uations felt to require high-dose SAIDs are chronic, or at least they persist for long periods. Consequently, SAID side effects become a major consideration and often lead to further empirical trials of nonsteroidal immunosuppressive agents, searching for a "steroid-sparing" effect, even when the SAID is apparently effective. Furthermore, dosage schedules aimed at minimizing side effects may have to take precedence over suppression of symptoms when high-dose SAIDs seem to be required for long periods.

Classic examples of situations requiring long-term, high-dose SAIDs include the nephritis of systemic lupus erythematosus, polymyositis, and several forms of systemic vasculitis, especially giant-cell arteritis. The rules here are not as simple as for the use of lower doses, but a few can be formulated. Although it is usually wise to begin with daily therapy, tapering to every other day may be attempted as soon as possible in order to minimize side effects. Assuming the basic disease process remains under good control, it may be possible to gradually change from 60 mg of prednisone every day to 120 mg every other day over the period of a few weeks. Once the disease process is under good control with every-other-day therapy, a gradual withdrawal usually should be attempted. For most diseases or manifestations, reductions of 10–20 mg every two to four weeks can be tried, and perhaps smaller decrements attempted after the every-other-day dose reaches the 60-mg range. If withdrawal cannot be achieved because of worsening of the manifestation being treated, a search for a "steroid-sparing" agent might be launched. Symptoms such as arthralgias often become a problem with infrequent dosage schedules and relatively rapid withdrawal, but these can often be managed with analgesics or NSAIDs if they are not contraindicated.

Very short courses of very high doses of systemic SAIDs have been called **steroid pulse therapy**. Usually about 1 gm/day of methyl-prednisolone is given intravenously for three days. There are anecdotal reports of this practice resulting in sustained benefits in patients with systemic lupus, rheumatoid arthritis, and a few other rheumatic diseases, with a minimum of serious side effects, but it is of unproven value, and a few cases of serious toxicity have been reported. Perhaps steroid pulse therapy is most often used in desperate situations such as the most serious forms of CNS lupus or the life-threatening manifestations of a systemic vasculitis. If such a program is to be used, it should usually be followed by a regular daily program of high-dose SAIDs.

Contraindications to the Use of Systemic SAIDs

Since systemic SAIDs should be used only when absolutely necessary, the only real contraindication to their use is the lack of an indication. Furthermore these agents cannot be abruptly withdrawn when a presumed side effect occurs. The risk of adrenal insufficiency and a flare in the underlying disease process is too great. In fact, if the presumed side effect is serious, the dose may have to be increased to match maximal adrenal SAID output under stress.

The list of rheumatic diseases and their manifestations that are **not** indications for systemic SAID therapy is lengthy (Table 3-6). Perhaps the most important is undiagnosed disease; an ill-defined rheumatic syndrome should be treated with SAIDs only under the most desperate of circumstances. With the possible exception of polymyalgia rheumatica, diagnostic-therapeutic trials of SAIDs are al-

Table 3-6. Common rheumatic disorders not requiring or benefitting from systemic SAID therapy

Osteoarthritis in any form

Degenerative disk disease in any form

Tendinitis, bursitis, enthesopathies

Fibromyalgia (fibrositis)

Spondyloarthropathies (unless NSAIDs are contraindicated)

Arthropathies due to infectious agents

Raynaud's phenomenon

Scleroderma syndromes (unless associated with inflammatory myopathy)

Osteonecrosis

most always doomed to failure and frequently prolong the diagnostic process. The diagnosis of a disease does not itself necessarily represent an indication for SAID therapy. Many patients with systemic lupus erythematosus, Sjögren's syndrome, mixed connective tissue disease, and hypersensitivity vasculitis will never require corticosteroids, nor will most patients with rheumatoid arthritis. Other common rheumatic disorders not requiring SAID therapy are listed in Table 3-6.

Clinical Aspects of Side Effects

With sustained use, SAID side effects are inevitable, but some individuals seem to be more susceptible than others, often for reasons that are not clear. In general the likelihood of any side effect becoming clinically apparent is a function of the total SAID dose used and the duration of therapy. Increased susceptibility to a side effect might simply reflect the pretreatment state of the target tissue; for example, a patient who already has postmenopausal osteoporosis will appear to be more susceptible to the effects of these agents on bone. Hypoalbuminemia has been associated with increased side effects, and this condition may actually indicate a reduction in the usual dosage. Concomitant use of certain drugs such as the barbiturates and rifampin may result in accelerated steroid metabolism and appear to reduce the side effects, but they also reduce beneficial effects. Side effects can be intentionally minimized by using infrequent (every-other-day) dosage schedules and, of course, by using the lowest possible SAID dose for the shortest possible time. Otherwise it has been suggested that a high-protein diet, calcium supplementation, and vigorous physical activity can help minimize some of the side effects. Some will almost always occur, however, and it is appropriate to point out here that the five-year mortality of naturally occurring untreated Cushing's syndrome is in excess of 50%.

SAID side effects result from a wide variety of pharmacologic actions, including negative nitrogen balance, immunosuppression, anti-inflammatory effects, and hypothalamic-pituitary-adrenal suppression. They are summarized in Table 3-7. Electrolyte disturbances, edema, hypertension, sexual dysfunction, hirsutism, striae, and plethora are more common in naturally occurring Cushing's syndrome or with the use of agents with mineralocorticoid activity. Others such as cataracts, glaucoma, pancreatitis, and aseptic necrosis of bone are more common in the iatrogenic syndrome. Of course, suppression of the hypothalamic-pituitary-adrenal axis usually results from systemic SAID therapy. The more important side effects listed in Table 3-7 will be discussed individually.

BODY HABITUS

The typical body habitus of the SAID-treated patient is well known and is usually a major concern to the patient, who may already be concerned with his or her body self-image. Weight gain is probably the most preventable aspect of the problem, but prevention may require vigorous dietary restrictions. A high-protein, low-carbohy-

Table 3-7. Summary of systemic SAID side effects

Body habitus
  Obesity—primarily central
  Growth retardation in children
CNS
  Benign intracranial hypertension
  Irritability
  Insomnia
  "Steroid psychosis"
Gastrointestinal
  Fatty liver
  Gastric hemorrhage
  Pancreatitis
  Peptic ulcer disease
Hematopoietic
  Lymphocytopenia
  Neutrophilic leukocytosis
Host defense
  Increased susceptibility to infection
  Masking infection (anti-inflammatory effect)
  Poor wound healing
Localized lipohypertrophy
  Aseptic necrosis of epiphyseal bone from medullary lipohypertrophy
  Epidural lipomatosis leading to cord compression
  Mediastinal lipomatosis
  Moon facies and "buffalo hump"
Metabolic-endocrine-renal
  Edema
  Hirsutism
  Hyperlipidemia predisposing to atherogenesis
  Hypertension
  Hypokalemia
  Hypothalamic-pituitary-adrenal axis suppression predisposing to
    addisonian crisis
  Impotence perhaps related to low serum testosterone levels
  Insulin resistance leading to diabetes mellitus
  Menstrual irregularities
Musculoskeletal
  Joint effusions
  Myopathy
  Osteoporosis
  Tendon ruptures
Skin
  Acne
  Fragility/ecchymosis
  Striae
"Steroid pseudorheumatism"
  Arthralgias/myalgias
  Systemic symptoms

drate diet has been thought to be beneficial. The problem is magnified in children and adolescents by SAID-induced early epiphyseal closure leading to growth retardation or even dwarfism. Infrequent dosage schedules may help minimize the problem.

CNS

Many patients treated with even low-dose SAIDs will complain of irritability and insomnia; often these symptoms improve with continued use and time. At the extreme end of this spectrum is the syndrome of "steroid psychosis"—a serious polymorphous psychiatric syndrome. The syndrome usually develops within a few days of beginning or escalating to high-dose therapy and has rarely been reported with less than the equivalent of 30 mg/day of prednisone. Since it is often not possible to withdraw SAID therapy, the manifestations can frequently be managed with haloperidol or a similar antipsychotic agent. Tricyclic antidepressant drugs have been noted to worsen the manifestations even when they are affective in nature. A small experience suggests that lithium may have a prophylactic effect.

EYES

Posterior subcapsular cataracts due to SAID therapy appear to occur more often in children, though this side effect was originally reported in adults with rheumatoid arthritis. In one survey cataracts were found in 29% of asthmatic children treated systemically for a year or longer. Alternate-day programs may minimize the risk.

GASTROINTESTINAL

Upper gastrointestinal bleeding has been reported in patients receiving short courses of high-dose SAIDs, suggesting that these agents predispose to the development of and bleeding from stress-related gastric injury. This observation might constitute an additional indication for prophylaxis with sucralfate or H_2-blocking agents under these circumstances. The role of systemic SAIDs in inducing peptic ulcer disease is less certain, and it has been suggested that daily doses of 20 mg of prednisone or less do not; however, it is likely that SAIDs interfere with healing of a pre-existing ulcer and probably predispose to hemorrhage. SAID-related fatty changes in the liver are common and should be considered in treated patients with hepatomegaly or mildly abnormal liver tests.

HEMATOPOIETIC

Other than their effects on circulating cells responsible for host defense activities, the hematologic changes resulting from SAID therapy have no clinical consequences; however, under certain circumstances they may be confusing. SAIDs regularly cause lymphocytopenia and eosinophilopenia, but their demarginating effect on granulocytes may lead to inappropriate searches for infection. A dramatic rise in the polymorphonuclear leukocyte count may occur as early as the first day of therapy with high doses, and though the counts tend to fall toward normal with continued treatment, they typically remain abnormally high even if SAID dosages are reduced. Total white blood cell counts in the range of 15,000–20,000/mm^3 are fairly common; however, rarely more than 6% band forms or toxic granulation are present.

HOST DEFENSE

Because of their immunosuppressive and anti-inflammatory effects, systemic SAIDs not only predispose to infection but also mask it. The immunosuppressive effect begins to become detectable with as little as 10–15 mg/day of prednisone, and as the dosage increases beyond that level, susceptibility to infection increases proportionally. At higher doses opportunistic infections become more prominent. Even lower doses may predispose to herpetic and yeast infections. A long-standing concern has been reactivation of pulmonary tuberculosis. Though this appears to happen infrequently, skin testing or a chest film prior to therapy has been recommended. Fortunately SAIDs exert only a weak antipyretic effect, and fever during the course of therapy is the usual clue to infection. Other expected physical and radiographic signs may be minimal due to the anti-inflammatory effect of these agents. Consequently fever, even in an otherwise asymptomatic patient, must be intensively investigated.

LOCALIZED LIPOHYPERTROPHY

Localized lipohypertrophy is responsible for the typical moon face and "buffalo hump" of SAID-treated patients, and occasionally mediastinal lipohypertrophy causes a confusing mediastinal mass on the chest film, though the nature of the mass can usually be resolved with computed tomography. Epidural lipohypertrophy has resulted in a number of cases of spinal cord compression and should be considered in any treated patient who develops signs of myelopathy.

The most common serious problem resulting from lipohypertrophy reflects this process in the bone marrow in or adjacent to epiphyseal bone. Because of the rising intramedullary pressure, the circulation is compromised, leading to necrosis of epiphyseal bone. This phenomenon can occur at any site but is most often symptomatic in the femoral and humeral heads, and it may occur simultaneously at multiple sites. Just how much SAIDs are required to produce this effect has been debated, but it has been reported to correlate better with short courses of high doses than with prolonged therapy. In the femoral head especially, it might be important to make an early diagnosis. Considerable experience has suggested that healing often occurs if the medullary hypertension is relieved surgically prior to bone collapse.

METABOLIC/ENDOCRINE

Mineralocorticoid and androgenic effects of prednisone and other synthetic SAIDs should be minimal to absent; yet they occur, perhaps because of actions that are not fully understood. It is possible that the impotence and menstrual irregularities associated with SAID use reflect, in part, consequences of the disease being treated rather than a side effect of these agents. Considerable evidence associates long-term SAID therapy, even in low doses, with clinically important atherogenicity, perhaps because of the hypercholesterolemic effect. The overall impact of these agents on lipids is complex and not yet fully defined.

Suppression of the hypothalamic-pituitary-adrenal axis by exogenous SAIDs has been extensively investigated. Even low doses can be shown to exert an effect within a few days; when high doses have been used, evidence of hypothalamic-pituitary-adrenal suppression may be detectable up to a year after withdrawal. The clinical consequences of this effect may have been exaggerated. Addisonian crises are rarely encountered; however, it is still universally recommended that approaches aimed at preventing such a crisis be undertaken. Either the status of the axis should be formally tested and proven normal or adequate replacement should be provided during periods of physical stress such as major surgery or trauma in anyone at potential risk for an addisonian crisis. Adequate replacement consists of maximal adrenal output under stressful situations—about 300 mg/day of hydrocortisone.

It can be debated whether SAIDs actually cause diabetes mellitus or simply unmask the underlying disease. In either event, hyperglycemia, even with ketosis, is frequently encountered with the higher doses. In patients with known diabetes, increased insulin requirements can be expected, and control may prove very difficult during periods of dose adjustment.

MUSCULOSKELETAL

Since its major manifestations are musculoskeletal, the SAID withdrawal syndrome, or "steroid pseudorheumatism" will be mentioned here. This is a frequently confounding collection of symptoms that occurs after abrupt cessation of SAID therapy. Within hours or at most a few days of the last dose, the patient develops myalgias, arthralgias, malaise, and a depressed feeling. The syndrome may persist for hours or a few days but responds dramatically to reinstitution of SAID therapy. A similar phenomenon has been reported to recur regularly in patients receiving high-dose SAIDs at infrequent intervals. In this case the withdrawal syndrome may mimic the disease being treated and is sometimes severe enough to justify a more frequent dosage schedule.

Steroid myopathy is a syndrome of predominantly proximal muscle weakness presumably related to the histologic finding of type 2 fiber atrophy; except for increased creatine excretion, no biochemical correlates exist. The syndrome occurs most often with the fluorinated compounds and may be more common in patients with polymyositis where it can be especially confounding. A vigorous exercise program may be partly prophylactic or even therapeutic.

Osteoporosis is an expected result of long-term, high-dose SAID therapy and has also been associated with low-dose therapy. Trabecular bone is predominantly affected, leading to vertebral body and rib fractures as the major symptomatic manifestations. Pretreatment bone mass influences the likelihood of significant clinical consequences. Recent studies have suggested little impact of low-dose SAIDs over a two-year period on the bone mass of women with rheumatoid arthritis, but the disease itself is associated with osteoporosis. Infrequent dosage schedules have not been shown to reduce the incidence or severity of the problem. Vitamin D supplementation has yielded conflicting results, and its use is controversial as either a prophylactic or therapeutic approach. Vigorous physical activity and adequate calcium intake are recommended. Calcitonin is of no proven value.

SKIN

Numerous cutaneous manifestations result from regular SAID therapy and are frequently the major side effect of concern to the patient. The skin thins, bruises easily, and lacerates with minor trauma. Poor wound healing magnifies the problem and may exaggerate the resulting scars. A fine sandpaper-like rash or folliculitis called **steroid acne** occurs commonly on the face and trunk. Because they persist after withdrawal of therapy, the striae may be the most distressing cutaneous side effect and they may be widespread. These cutaneous effects contribute to the negative body image problem experienced by many patients.

Bibliography

BASIC PHARMACOLOGY

Allison, A. C., and Lee, S. W. The mode of action of anti-rheumatic drugs. 1. Anti-inflammatory and immunosuppressive effects of gluco-corticoids. *Prog. Drug. Res.* 33:63–81, 1989.

Beato, M., et al. Gene regulation by steroid hormones. *J. Steroid Biochem.* 27:9–14, 1987.

Black, H. E. The effects of steroids upon the gastrointestinal tract. *Toxicol. Pathol.* 16:213–222, 1988.

Claman, H. N. Glucocorticosteroids I, II: Anti-inflammatory mechanisms, the clinical responses. *Hosp. Pract.* 18:123–134, 143–151, 1983.

Dale, M. M., and Foreman, J. C. (eds.). *Textbook of Immunopharmacology* Oxford: Blackwell, 1989.

Goodwin, J. S. Mechanism of action of glucocorticosteroids. *J. Clin. Invest.* 77:1244–1250, 1986.

Oikarinen, A. I., Uitto, J., and Oikarinen, J. Glucocorticoid action on connective tissue: from molecular mechanisms to clinical practice. *Med. Biol.* 64:221–230, 1986.

Peers, S. H., and Flower, R. J. The role of lipocortin in corticosteroid actions. *Am. Rev. Respir. Dis.* 141:S18–21, 1990.

Persson, C. G. A., and Pipkorn, U. Glucocorticoids. *Chem. Immunol.* 49:264–277, 1990.

Rugstad, H. E. Antiinflammatory and immunoregulatory effects of glucocorticoids: mode of action. *Scand. J. Rheumatol.* 76(suppl):257–264, 1988.

Scheimer, R. P., Claman, H. N., and Oronsky, A. (eds.). *Anti-inflammatory Steroid Action.* Orlando: Academic, 1989.

Synder, F. Biochemistry of platelet-activating factor: A unique class of biologically active phospholipids (42839). *Proc. Soc. Exp. Biol. Med.* 190:125–135, 1988.

Thompson, E. B. The structure of the human glucocorticoid receptor and its gene. *J. Steroid Biochem.* 27:105–108, 1987.

CLINICAL INDICATIONS

Axelrod, L. Glucocorticoids. In W. N. Kelley et al (eds.), *Textbook of Rheumatology* (3rd ed.). Philadelphia: Saunders, 1989. Pp. 845–861.

Behrens, T. W., and Goodwin, J. S. Glucocorticoids. In D. J. McCarty (ed.), *Arthritis and Allied Conditions* (11th ed.). Philadelphia: Lea & Febiger, 1989. Pp. 604–621.

Bergrem, H., and Refvem O. K. Altered prednisolone pharmacokinetics in patients treated with rifampicin. *Acta Med. Scand.* 213:339–343, 1983.

Buchanan, W. W., Stephen, L. J., and Buchanan, H. M. Are 'homeopathic' doses of oral corticosteroids effective in rheumatoid arthritis? *Clin. Exp. Rheumatol.* 6:281–284, 1988.

Claman, H. N. Anti-inflammatory Effects of Corticosteroids. In M. S. Mitchell and J. L. Fahey (eds.), *Clinics in Immunology and Allergy* (Vol. 4). Philadelphia: Saunders, 1984. Pp. 317–329.

Empire Rheumatism Council. Multi-centre controlled trial comparing cortisone acetate and acetyl salicylic acid in the long-term treatment of rheumatoid arthritis. *Ann. Rheum. Dis.* 16:277–289, 1957.

Garber, E. K., Fan, P. T., and Bluestone, R. Realistic guidelines of corticosteroid therapy in rheumatic disease. *Semin. Arthritis Rheum.* 11:231–256, 1981.

Gray, R. G., and Gottlieb, N. L. Intra-articular corticosteroids. *Clin. Orthop.* 177:235–263, 1983.

Harris, E. D. Jr., et al. Low dose prednisolone therapy in rheumatoid arthritis: a double-blind study. *J. Rheumatol.* 10:713–721, 1983.

Iglehart, I. W., et al. Intravenous pulsed steroids in rheumatoid arthritis: A comparative dose study. *J. Rheumatol.* 17:159–162, 1990.

Kehrl, J. H., and Fauci, A. S. The clinical use of glucocorticoids. *Ann. Allergy* 50:2–8, 1983.

Nelson, A. M., and Conn, D. L. Glucocorticoids in rheumatic disease. *Mayo Clin. Proc.* 55:758–769, 1980.

SIDE EFFECTS

Cogan, M. G., et al. Prevention of prednisone-induced negative nitrogen balance. *Ann. Intern. Med.* 95:158–161, 1981.

Conn, H. O., and Poynard, T. Adrenocorticosteroid administration and peptic ulcer: A critical analysis. *J. Chronic Dis.* 38:457–468, 1985.

Gallant, C., and Kenny, P. Oral glucocorticoids and their complications. *J. Am. Acad. Dermatol.* 14:161–177, 1986.

George, W. E., Jr., et al. Medical management of steroid-induced epidural lipomatosis. *N. Engl. J. Med.* 308:316–319, 1983.

Gray, R. E., et al. A double-blind study of deflazacort and prednisone in patients with chronic inflammatory disorders. *Arthritis Rheum.* 34:287–295, 1991.

Hall, R. C. W., et al. Presentation of the steroid psychoses. *J. Nerv. Ment. Dis.* 167:229–236, 1979.

Horber, F. F., et al. Thigh muscle mass and function in patients treated with glucocorticoids. *Eur. J. Clin. Invest.* 15:302–307, 1985.

Kahl, L., and Medsger, T. A., Jr. Severe arthralgias after wide fluctuation in corticosteroid dosage. *J. Rheumatol.* 13:1063–1065, 1986.

Lally, E. V. High-dose corticosteroid therapy: Association with noninflammatory synovial effusions. *Arthritis Rheum.* 26:1283–1287, 1983.

Lukert, B. P., and Raisz, L. G. Glucocorticoid-induced osteoporosis: Pathogenesis and management. *Ann. Intern. Med.* 112:352–364, 1990.

MacAdams, M. R., White, R. H., and Chipps, B. E. Reduction of serum testosterone levels during chronic glucocorticoid therapy. *Ann. Intern. Med.* 104:648–651, 1986.

Messer, J., et al. Association of adrenocorticosteroid therapy and peptic-ulcer disease. *N. Engl. J. Med.* 309:21–24, 1983.

Piper, J. M., Ray W. A., Daugherty, M. S., and Griffin, M. R. Corticosteroid use and peptic ulcer disease: role of nonsteroidal anti-inflammatory drugs. *Ann. Intern. Med.* 114:735–740, 1991.

Sambrook, P. N., et al. Effects of low dose corticosteroids on bone mass in rheumatoid arthritis: a longitudinal study. *Ann. Rheum. Dis.* 48:535–538, 1989.

Taskinen, M. R., et al. Short-term effects of prednisone on serum lipids and high density lipoprotein subfractions in normolipidemic healthy men. *J. Clin. Endocrinol. Metab.* 67:291–294, 1988.

4

Slow-Acting Antirheumatic Drugs (Including Immunosuppressive Agents)

Included in this chapter are a diverse group of agents with demonstrated antirheumatic effects, primarily in rheumatoid arthritis (RA); however, several, including the immunosuppressive agents, are widely used for other rheumatic disorders. Although the group is quite heterogeneous and has no recognized common mechanism of action, its members are clearly not corticosteroids or nonsteroidal anti-inflammatory drugs (NSAIDs). They do share the common feature of acting relatively slowly, over weeks to months, at least in patients with RA. These drugs have been studied most intensively in that disease and the emphasis here will be on their role in managing it, but other indications also will be addressed. The agents composing this group are listed in Table 4-1. A minimum requirement for inclusion is an adequate number (at least two) of double-blind controlled trials in RA documenting significant efficacy over a period of at least several months.

The Concept of Slow-Acting Drug Therapy in RA

The drugs listed in Table 4-1 are often referred to as **second-line agents**, the **first-line agents** being the NSAIDs. The implication is that they are to be used only after the NSAIDs have failed, but the decision to begin one of these drugs is usually more complex than that. **Disease modifying antirheumatic drug [DMARD]** is another term frequently used to refer to this group, but disease modification is a very difficult action to prove. **Remittive** has also been used in reference to these drugs, but they do not usually result in a complete clinical remission. Hence, for lack of a better term, **slow-acting** (SAARDs) will be the one employed here, even though some of the agents on the list may exert an effect in weeks instead of months.

Other than regarding their basic pharmacology and onset of action, it is difficult to define just how these drugs differ from the NSAIDs and the corticosteroids. It is generally felt that the latter do not alter outcome in patients with RA, but simply suppress inflammation and symptoms on a day-to-day basis. To prove that a drug alters outcome in RA would require a prolonged, perhaps a decade, placebo-controlled trial, and such a study has not been and probably never will be done. Furthermore no general agreement exists on how to measure outcome even if it were feasible to try to do so. Nonetheless many, if not most, clinical rheumatologists feel that these slow-acting agents can favorably modify outcome in RA, and

Table 4-1. Slow-acting antirheumatic drugs

FDA approved for use in RA
Parenteral gold salts
  Gold sodium thiomalate (Myochrysine)—50 mg/ml
  Gold sodium thioglucose (Solganal)—50 mg/ml

Oral gold salts
  Auranofin (Ridaura)—3 mg

D-penicillamine
  (Depen, Cuprimine)—125, 250 mg

Azathioprine
  (Imuran)—50 mg

Antimalarials
  Chloroquine* (Aralen)—250, 500 mg
  Hydroxychloroquine (Plaquenil)—200 mg

Methotrexate
  Rheumatrex—2.5 mg (and 25 mg/ml)

Not (yet) FDA approved for use in RA
Sulfasalazine* (Azulfidine)—500 mg

Cyclophosphamide (Cytoxan)—25, 50 mg

(?) Cyclosporin (Sandimmune)—100 mg/ml (PO solution)

*Available generically.

hence really are DMARDs; this discussion will proceed as if that were true.

What has been documented in the controlled trials of these agents is that they gradually modify disease activity to a greater degree than the NSAIDs had done. Consequently they can be considered useful only in patients with persistent disease activity. Signs and symptoms of disease activity include joint pain, especially at rest, prolonged morning stiffness, fatigue, and tender and swollen joints on physical examination. In the laboratory, elevated acute-phase reactants (or increased erythrocyte sedimentation rate) and the anemia of chronic disease also suggest disease activity. Probably the single most reliable indicator is the number of tender and swollen joints. It should be remembered, however, that all of these findings can be suppressed by corticosteroid therapy, but the true need for such therapy could itself be considered an indicator of disease activity.

The toxicity of the SAARDs may, on the average, actually be no greater than that of the NSAIDs, but they are widely perceived as being more dangerous. Toxicity monitoring of some type is considered necessary for all of these agents, and that adds to their expense and to patient inconvenience. Consequently it is obviously best not to use these agents unless they are needed, and not all patients with RA need them.

The general recommendation that they be prescribed for patients who have failed to respond to NSAIDs is overly simplistic. The decision to begin slow-acting therapy is heavily influenced by apparent disease severity. In patients with long-standing disease, severity is easy to assess, but it is just these signs of severe disease that one wishes to prevent; therefore, it would be useful to be able to predict severe disease early in its course and select those patients with signs of a poor prognosis for more aggressive therapy. Fortunately several prognostic indicators, which may be present early in the course of RA, suggest an unfavorable outcome. These include widespread active disease (12 or more joints simultaneously inflamed), subcutaneous nodules, strongly positive test for rheumatoid factor (RF), and early appearance of destructive changes on joint radiographs. For a patient with none of these signs early in the course of the disease, it might be wise to continue to try various NSAIDs more or less indefinitely before making a slow-acting drug commitment. Conversely, for a patient who has any of them in the first year or two of the disease, it might be desirable to begin slow-acting therapy early, even if the patient is relatively comfortable taking only salicylates.

Despite the heterogeneity of the group, the SAARDs tend to share a number of common features, especially in the context of their use in RA. Perhaps the most disconcerting common feature is their mechanism of action in RA, which is unknown or poorly understood for all of them. Although a number of pharmacologic actions have been identified for all of these drugs, in most cases no one or combination of them is sufficient to fully explain their effects on the disease. The beneficial effects of many of these agents were discovered serendipitously. As already implied for most of these drugs, it takes several months—at least two—before any beneficial effects become apparent, and several more months of therapy—at least six total—are required before any one drug can be declared a failure.

On the average a satisfactory therapeutic response can be expected in only slightly more than half of the treated patients, but some drugs are more predictably effective than others. Response to one drug does not necessarily predict response to another, so that a sequential trial of three or four agents should result in a satisfactory response in the large majority of the population. Depending on the drug, 10–20% or more of treated patients will stop it in the first six months of therapy because of side effects. Adverse responses to one drug do not necessarily predict adverse responses to another, so that again sequential trials should result in the identification of a tolerable agent.

Toxicity tends to parallel efficacy. Much of the expense involved in the use of these agents derives from toxicity monitoring. Consequently the more likely a drug is to be effective, the more expensive it tends to be. Considering both failure to respond and toxicity, only about half of the patients treated with any one agent will continue to take it beyond one year; however, many of the patients continuing to take the drug will discontinue it later because of late toxicity or apparent loss of efficacy.

None of these agents induces a permanent remission or cure; therefore, if it is discontinued in a patient who seems to be responding, the disease activity can be expected to return gradually. No finite predefined courses are established for the SAARDs; although there

Table 4-2. Proposed mechanisms of immunoglobulin reduction by SAARDs

Agent	Mechanism
Azathioprine, 6-mercaptopurine	↓ B cell function and numbers
Chloroquine	↓ Lymphocyte proliferation (↓ IL-1) ↓ Macrophage antigen processing ↓ B-memory antigen processing
(Cyclophosphamide, chlorambucil)	↓ B cell proliferation
Gold compounds	↓ B cell proliferation (↓ IL-1)
Methotrexate	↓ Lymphocyte proliferation (↓ IL-1) ↓ Macrophage activation
Sulfasalazine	↓ Lymphocyte (B) proliferation?
(Levamisole)	↑ T suppressor function?
(Cyclosporin)	↓ Lymphocyte proliferation (↓ IL-2)
NSAIDs	↑ T suppressor function (↓ PGE$_2$)
SAIDs	↓ Lymphocyte proliferation (↓ IL-1) ↑ Fractional catabolism immunoglobulins ↓ Circulating T-lymphocytes (especially T-helper) ↓ Lymphoid mass (catabolic effect)

Key: (   ), not yet approved by FDA for use in RA; IL, interleukin; NSAIDs, nonsteroidal anti-inflammatory drugs; PG, prostaglandin; SAARDs, slow-acting anti-rheumatic drugs; SAIDs, steroidal anti-inflammatory drugs.

are unsuccessful trials, successful therapy is usually continued indefinitely. Lack of long-term or cumulative toxicity is, therefore, a desirable attribute in one of these agents. Ongoing NSAID and corticosteroid therapy is continued as long as needed after beginning a slow-acting agent. Hopefully at least the corticosteroids can be withdrawn later after a response to the SAARD becomes apparent.

The recognized mechanisms of the drugs to be discussed under SAARDs are highly varied. The mechanisms range from cytotoxicity, induced by cross-linking of DNA or by reduced availability of purines for DNA synthesis, sometimes with inhibition of RNA and protein synthesis, to decreases in receptors or increases in free sulfhydryl groups on macromolecules. Some drugs have highly theoretical mechanisms; others are well established, although even for the latter it is often unclear that the well-established mechanisms are the ones responsible for the drugs' utility as SAARDs. For each member or group, the accepted mechanisms will be presented, and an attempt will be made to relate the mechanism to the proposed utility in RA.

As previously stated, one aspect the SAARDs have in common, in addition to alleviating symptoms and possibly progression of the disease, is a slow onset of effect. Despite differing initial SAARD mechanisms, they may also have another feature in common, i.e., one end mechanism. In tabulating the effects of SAARDs, it becomes apparent that effects in many systems are opposite directions; however, the vast majority, and possibly all, of the SAARDs ultimately result in decreased levels of immunoglobulins, particularly IgG. The purpose in pointing this out is only to declare it, **not** to state categorically, and perhaps foolishly, that this is indeed how all SAARDs act; however, such an observation is highly intriguing (and suggestive), especially in view of the wide acceptance of RA as an autoimmune disease. Indeed, the observation is interesting enough that it should be kept in mind as the reader reviews the data for the individual agents.

As a perhaps prejudicial introduction, but more so to put the data together in an opportune place, the individual agents to be discussed are listed in Table 4-2 together with the proposed mechanism(s) whereby decreases in immunoglobulin(s) are effected. Data for two drugs, levamisole and sulfasalazine, are incomplete. Included in the list are two categories of drugs covered in previous sections, namely the NSAIDs (Chapter 2) and the steroidal anti-inflammatory drugs (SAIDs; Chapter 3). Both have been noted to have some immunomodulatory effects, specifically the ability to lower immunoglobulins. For NSAIDs, the effect may be rapid and relatively small. For SAIDs, immunomodulatory effects are slow to develop, and SAIDs could thus even be considered together with SAARDs; their distinguishing anti-inflammatory effects, which develop much more quickly, justify their consideration alone, however. The reader is referred to the appropriate chapters for additional details of the actions of NSAIDs and SAIDs.

Specific Agents

Gold Compounds

In the 1920s it was widely believed that RA was tuberculous in nature, and there was some enthusiasm for experimenting with the salts of gold and other heavy metals in tuberculosis, real or imagined. Gold salts were first used in RA in 1927, and the apparent success of the therapy inspired Forestier to use it in over 500 patients. He reported his experience in the 1930s, and, as a result, various forms of chrysotherapy came into vogue, but very large doses were often used and it rapidly became apparent that serious toxicity was a major limiting factor. Chrysotherapy continued to be controversial until the British Empire Rheumatism Council published their carefully done double-blind and placebo-controlled study in the early 1960s. This was the first study to clearly document efficacy, and it established the relative safety of modest doses given in a gradual fashion. Modern dosage schedules are derived from this study, and attempts to modify them in various ways have generally failed to demonstrate any advantages over the original program.

Two parenteral gold preparations are available in this country: gold sodium thiomalate (GSTM) (Myochrysine) in a water vehicle and gold sodium thioglucose (GSTG) (Solganal) in a sesame oil vehicle. Both are 50% gold by weight and are intended only for intramuscular administration. The two agents can be used interchangeably in the same dosage schedule. GSTM is easier to give but is more rapidly absorbed and is associated with postinjection reactions. GSTG is more difficult to administer and is more painful but causes few postinjection reactions presumably because of its more gradual absorption. Many clinicians elect to begin with GSTM and then change to GSTG if postinjection reactions occur. The cost of the two preparations is similar and is not based on the market price of elemental gold. Each 50-mg injection contains about $0.30 worth of the metal.

Auranofin was intentionally designed as an absorbable gold compound to be used in RA as an alternative to parenteral chrysotherapy. It was hoped that the resulting lower and more sustained blood levels would minimize toxicity without interfering with efficacy. As it turns out, it is not certain that auranofin is really an oral equivalent of parenteral gold. The two agents differ in many ways, and it is apparent that auranofin is both less toxic and less effective than the parenteral compounds. They should not be regarded as interchangeable agents. Auranofin is available in 3-mg capsules and is marketed only as Ridaura.

BASIC PHARMACOLOGY

General Properties

In some contrast to perceived therapeutic differences, the parenterally administered gold compounds and the orally administered gold compound auranofin are much more similar than dissimilar at the cellular level. To avoid repetition, the general features of gold compounds are covered without discrimination as to parenteral versus oral administration routes. The few features that are unique to either the parenteral compounds or to auranofin are pointed out in the sections that follow.

The clinically useful gold compounds all contain an aurothiol (gold mercaptide) group. The structures of three clinically used gold compounds are shown in Fig. 4-1 for reference. The binding of monovalent gold in this chemical group is **not** really salt-like (association of highly ionized participants by charge attraction, little electron sharing in a true bond), but rather is more covalent in nature (some electron sharing in the bond). The aurothiol group in auranofin is the least ionic and most stable, due to the additional interaction of its aurothiol with triethylphosphorous.

The chemical stability of auranofin accounts in part for its oral efficacy; however, this same stability, combined with low ($\approx$ 25%) absorption, partly due to its gastrointestinal side effects, may also account for its possibly decreased in vivo efficacy compared with parenteral compounds.

The three gold compounds in use are all water soluble, but to different degrees. Auranofin has the least water solubility and the greatest lipid solubility, in part a result of the esterification of all available hydroxyl groups on the glucose cycle. The parenterally used compounds can be administered as soluble preparations in aqueous vehicles or as insoluble suspensions in oil vehicles.

Administration of auranofin in its usual daily regimen, or of parenteral preparations at weekly intervals, reportedly produces max-

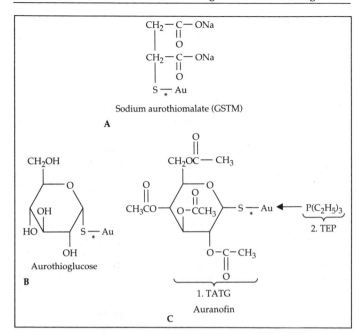

Fig. 4-1. Structures of gold compounds. A and B are parenterally used, whereas C is used by oral administration. In C, gold is doubly coordinated, to (1) tetra-acetylthioglucose (TATG) and (2) triethylphosphine (TEP). (*, aurothiol bond.)

imal levels in **approximately** the same time frame. The maximum levels attained by auranofin and the parenteral compounds differ and occur in this order:

parenteral, soluble > auranofin > parenteral, suspension

Since it appears that gold compounds may have biphasic effects in many systems, the actual levels attained and sustained could be critical features of therapy outcome: Levels that are continuously very low may not simply lack the desired therapeutic effect, but could also (**theoretically**) intensify some aspects. Perceived differences in therapeutic efficacy among the gold compounds may thus reflect differences in levels as a function of a combination of any or all of the following: the chemical nature of the compound, absorption rate/extent, side effect intolerance, and toxicity.

The gold moiety of the gold compounds apparently binds and exchanges to other sulfhydryl groups, first in blood, then on the surface of various cells (to be taken up or have effect, or both), and ultimately to intracellular groups. Intracellular distribution (and eventually elimination) also involves exchanges to various sulfhydryl groups. Distribution and accumulation (and redistribution/elimination) of gold compounds are very slow, and the distinct phases of mainly blood binding can be observed over days, weeks, and even months.

Drug half-lives are totally dose-dependent and are in the order of three months for all of them, although, due to greater accumulation with the parenteral forms, excretion can be detected up to a year after the last dose. Gold is excreted renally. This, together with kidney accumulation may predispose the kidney to toxic effects.

Coadministration of sulfhydryl reagents can prevent gold compound effects: Levels of free sulfhydryls in the circulation, which are notably low in RA, and the amount and types of intracellular sulfhydryls available, could thus regulate the effectiveness and toxicity of these drugs.

The mode of administration may determine the pattern and possibly the degree of distribution. Parenteral gold compounds administered as water-soluble preparations are rapidly and almost completely absorbed and circulate bound to plasma proteins, with the highest organ concentrations found in the kidney. Gold compounds administered as suspensions are slowly absorbed and significantly phagocytosed, particularly by the reticuloendothelial system; highest levels usually occur in the spleen and liver, but significant levels may also occur in the kidneys.

Active (and inactive) gold compounds all result in accumulation of gold in synovial cells and in cells of the kidney. The gold is found in cytoplasmic filaments or incorporated into characteristic structures known as **aurosomes** (modified lysosomes). Gold accumulation also occurs within the lysosomes of synovial macrophages. Inflamed joints accumulate significantly higher amounts of gold than do noninflamed joints; the greater accumulation may reflect in part the consequences of increased delivery, secondary to vascular changes, and also the higher populations of phagocytic cells.

Several consequences of the accumulation of gold/formation of aurosomes are probably localization/accumulation of gold at sites of inflammation as described before, long time-dependence for both accumulation and elimination, and occurrence of toxicity in other sites (kidney) of localization/accumulation of gold.

The function of three primary cell types, i.e., neutrophils, monocytes/macrophages, and lymphocytes, involved in inflammatory responses may be altered by gold compounds. Both the latter are mostly involved in the chronic states, whereas the former is involved in initiation as well as chronic stages. The mechanisms of action covered in subsequent sections are based mainly on data for two of the three available gold compounds, namely auranofin and GSTM, and much of the data discussed is from in vitro systems. Direct in vivo confirmation is often difficult or impossible, and there is a presumption that in vivo activity is at least qualitatively similar to activity in vitro.

Mechanisms of Antirheumatic Effects

Effects on Neutrophils

Until recently it was often stated that only auranofin had significant in vitro effects on the function of neutrophils. Specifically, auranofin (and other gold compounds) inhibits formation of leukotriene B_4 (LTB_4; see Chapter 1 for details of LTB_4 formation), phagocytosis, degranulation, and chemotaxis. The inhibitory effects occur to the greatest degree for stimuli that induce phagocytic responses.

Inhibition of LTB_4 production by gold compounds apparently does not involve direct effects on 5-lipoxygenase. The inhibition appears to occur at a step subsequent to protein kinase C involvement. Indeed, low concentrations of both auranofin and GSTM can indirectly (through phospholipase C activation) activate protein kinase C, an effect that should promote formation of eicosanoids, including LTB_4, but does not in intact systems. This is still an evolving area of investigation and additional details can be expected. The bottom line is important, however, and that is that all major functions of neutrophils can be significantly inhibited by auranofin and probably other gold compounds.

An explanation for the apparently weaker effects of GSTM in vitro on neutrophil functions has recently been offered and may apply to other cell populations as well. Most gold compound effects on individual cell functions are defined in in vitro systems, and thus the effect of the drug can be influenced by milieu composition. For example, neutrophil effects of GSTM are minimal without thiocyanate in the incubation mixture, whereas significant inhibition (of superoxide production) occurs when thiocyanate is included. The latter is attributed to formation of aurocyanide, presumed to be an active species also generated in vivo (up to 200 μM thiocyanate is present in plasma and can be converted to cyanide by neutrophils); exogenous aurocyanide was likewise inhibitory.

It has been argued that the dramatic inhibitory effects of gold compounds on neutrophils are not significantly involved in the efficacy of gold in rheumatoid therapy. This argument is based mainly on differences in time courses: Effects on neutrophils are very rapid, whereas clinical improvement is quite slow. Viewed as a multistep system, this could also be interpreted as effects on neutrophil contributions are not rate-limiting. In the latter case, effects on neutrophils could still contribute to the total effect once the rate-limiting step also came under control.

Effects on Monocytes/Macrophages

Details of the formation and effects of interleukin-1 (IL-1) have been presented previously under SAIDs; Chapter 3). This chapter should be consulted for additional details about the cytokines that are referred to in the following sections.

Monocytes and their tissue counterparts, macrophages, are active contributors to the inflammatory cascade. Monocytes are attracted to sites of inflammation and are activated by numerous stimuli, including products of neutrophils. Monocytes release LTB_4, PGE_2, IL-1, and more. Macrophages are similarly activated and release the same products. In addition, macrophages are involved in antibody processing and presentation. Macrophages are thus involved in humoral and cell-mediated immune responses, directly and through mediator effects.

Production of LTB_4 and IL-1 by monocytes and macrophages in vitro is inhibited by auranofin or GSTM. The effect on IL-1 is biphasic for both compounds (low doses stimulate, high doses inhibit). A slight difference exists between high-dose auranofin and high-dose GSTM: Auranofin inhibits levels of both released IL-1 and cell-associated IL-1, whereas GSTM inhibits released IL-1 only. IL-1 has potent inflammatory effects, stimulates synovial cells to release PGE_2 and collagenase, and also activates T-lymphocytes. The latter in turn release additional factors (e.g., IL-2) that bring other cells (e.g., B-lymphocytes) into play. Reduction in IL-1 can thus give anti-inflammatory and immunomodulatory results. Indeed, reduction in IL-1 is also a prominent mechanism of the SAIDs (Chapter 3).

Some data support the applicability of the in vitro effects on IL-1 to the in vivo situation. Large numbers of IL-1–positive cells are found in the blood of RA patients; even higher numbers of IL-1–positive cells are found in synovial fluid. Administration of parenteral gold does result in a significantly lower number of positive cells in the circulation and, presumably, in synovial fluid.

Gold compounds may also decrease leukocyte populations. Auranofin has recently been shown to decrease macrophage numbers and granulocyte colonies formed from precursor cells in vitro. These effects were observed at **very** low (nM) concentrations, but applicability to in vivo levels that might be reached in bone marrow, for example, are unclear.

Effects on Lymphocytes

Since T-lymphocytes are directly stimulated by IL-1, decreased levels of IL-1 can lead to decreased involvement of several dependent populations of lymphocytes. Proliferative responses of lymphocytes are reduced due to decreased IL-2; thus, fewer B- and T-lymphocytes may be present subsequent to gold therapy, and both humoral and cell-mediated immune responses may be reduced. In addition to indirect effects through the IL-1, IL-2 sequence, GSTM has been found to have direct inhibitory effects on B-lymphocytes.

Interferon (IFΓ; IF), primarily a product of T-helper lymphocytes (some also produced by T-suppressor and B-lymphocytes), is also reduced, at least at higher concentrations of gold (another example of concentration-dependent biphasic response). IF effects include inhibition of proliferation of many types of cells and complement fixation, as well as stimulation of phagocytosis, cytotoxicity, and PGE_2 production. Thus, the net of IF's various opposing effects, and thus of inhibition of IF formation, is difficult to predict.

Inhibition of B-lymphocyte proliferation and antibody formation can lead to decreased levels of immunoglobulins, including RF (in the circulation as well as in synovial fluid). Importantly, decreases in IgG, IgM, and IgA, including the corresponding RFs, have been observed as a result of gold therapy. It is possible that the slow onset of observable therapeutic effect reflects not only the time required to achieve adequate levels of gold at the appropriate sites, but also removal of cell populations and turnover/clearance of certain of their products, i.e., antibodies.

Other Effects

Angiogenesis is a notable feature of the joint inflammatory response in RA. Angiogenesis may be stimulated by factors released by monocytes/macrophages, including IL-1, acting on endothelial cells.

GSTM recently has been shown to inhibit growth supplement–induced proliferative responses of endothelial cells in culture. In addition, IFΓ-induced surface receptor expression was reduced by GSTM.

Activation of the complement cascade by several different paths occurs and contributes to the total joint inflammatory response, as described in previous chapters. Gold compounds interact rapidly with the complement component C1q, the initiation unit of the cascade, and thus can interfere with complement activation and dependent effects, i.e., leukocyte activation. Curiously, C1q subunits have significant homology with collagen at their N-termini. Since gold compounds can inhibit collagen degradation, it is tempting to speculate that this is accomplished by gold binding to collagen, although effect on metalloproteinases or collagenase, or both, is also a possibility. GSTM does not change elastin hydrolysis by monocytes in vitro directly or after in vivo drug administration.

Acute-phase or stress proteins have been noted to increase in response to gold therapy. Since stress proteins have a role in normal and reparative cellular processes, increases in them may represent an additional mechanism of antirheumatoid effect. Inhibitory effects of GSTM on (a) DNA polymerase (α) have been reported. The significance of this in the context of therapeutic efficacy is unclear.

As described earlier, gold compounds can interact with free sulfhydryls. Low free sulfhydryl levels occur in RA, which may be secondary to formation of disulfide bonds contained in immune complexes. This implies that sulfhydryl levels can be a measure of disease status. Importantly, gold therapy significantly increases free sulfhydryl levels and therefore is presumed to interfere with sulfhydryl-disulfide exchange reactions. It has been proposed that the lesser degree of in vivo immunoglobulin reduction obtained with auranofin reflects its lesser sulfhydryl reactivity. In addition to sulfhydryl levels, intracellular levels of metallothioneins (metal-binding proteins), which are inducible, may influence gold effects. Interference with sulfhydryl-disulfide exchange reactions is a proposed mechanism for D-penicillamine also (see D-Penicillamine).

Mechanisms of Side Effects and Drug Interactions

The dose-response relationship for therapeutic effects of gold is not well separated from the dose-response relationships for several common side effects, including pruritic rashes that may progress to exfoliative dermatitis, nephrotic syndrome, and, for auranofin, diarrhea. The human leukocyte antigen haplotype DR-3 (HLA-DR3) has been reported to predispose to development of side effects/toxicity. A relationship between presence of circulating antibodies to a peptide derived from a ribonucleoprotein and gold intolerance has also been suggested.

Overt cytotoxic effects of auranofin have been proposed and may occur through several mechanisms; some of these mechanisms also apply to other gold compounds. One mechanism that would be specific to auranofin is alkylation of sulfhydryl groups to which gold triethylphosphine attaches, with subsequent changes in structure and function of the original macromolecule. For all the gold compounds, the same type of sulfhydryl-disulfide exchange that can be beneficial could also occur with normal molecules, thus altering functional status and disrupting normal cellular processes. This is probably the mechanism whereby auranofin inhibits gastrointestinal transport adenosinetriphosphatase (ATPase), and possibly other membrane and mitochondrial transport processes. Consumption of glutathione (by gold binding) and prevention of its regeneration (by inhibition of involved enzymes) have been proposed to result in gold-induced lipid peroxidation. Increased lipid peroxidation could impact integrity of various membranes, e.g., the cytoskeleton, even resulting in cell death.

The precise mechanism of gold-induced proteinuria is not known but could involve any/all of the aforementioned. As noted previously, gold accumulation (aurosomes) in kidney cells is relatively common and gold is renally excreted. Low-level kidney damage also has been suggested to be common. For example, in one study, increased levels of urinary enzymes and increased tubular cell excretion were noted in gold NSAID–treated patients in the absence of otherwise-altered renal function. These changes were not observed in patients treated with NSAIDs only, which may indicate an effect of gold alone, or potentially an interaction of gold-NSAIDs. An interaction between gold and salicylates in altering liver function has been suggested but is not well documented. Administration of aspirin and gold together may result in increased hepatic enzyme levels.

Several of the side effects of gold therapy appear to have a hypersensitivity component, perhaps initiated by gold-altered macromolecules. A hypersensitivity origin would be consistent with the occurrence of eosinophilia. Hypersensitivity may be involved in skin symptoms and pneumonitis, and possibly leukopenia/thrombocytopenia. A case report of gold pneumonitis that responded only after additional removal of NSAID (naproxen) therapy suggests involvement of 5-lipoxygenase products, e.g., slow-reacting substance of anaphylaxis (SRS-A; leukotrienes) (see Aspirin Hypersensitivity, Chapter 2).

Because gold compounds can activate phospholipase C and thus theoretically promote formation of eicosanoids, it has been suggested that disease flares during therapy with gold may reflect the effects of increased PGE_2 in particular. On this basis, addition of NSAIDs has been used as a means of reducing flare occurrence. In view of the potential for interactions mentioned previously, additional data to support the safety of this combination would seem appropriate.

The diarrhea frequently seen with auranofin has been suggested to result in part from interference by gold with gastrointestinal transport ATPase activity. The latter supports secondary active uptake processes including bile salt reabsorption in the distal small bowel. The result of transport ATPase inhibition and decreased bile salt reabsorption would be increased bile salt levels in the large intestine, which would promote diarrhea. A small amount of gold is eliminated by biliary secretion, which could also increase gastrointestinal exposure and symptoms.

Gold, as other metals, forms complexes with dimercaprol (BAL), a sulfhydryl reagent. In acute, severe toxicity, clearance, and symptom reduction, can be accelerated by inclusion of BAL in the treatment regimen. D-penicillamine has been used in the treatment of heavy metal intoxication, but its specific use for gold toxicity is not of proven value.

PARENTERAL GOLD

Expectations and Dosage Schedules in RA

The parenteral gold salts are among the more effective and more toxic of the slow-acting agents. Over 50%, perhaps as many as 70%, of treated patients can expect a satisfactory therapeutic response, and the response rate **may** be even higher if the initial trial is extended beyond six months. Meanwhile about 15% of treated patients will discontinue therapy in the first six months because of side effects. No beneficial response is expected before about three months of therapy, and a cumulative total dose of at least 1 gm (about five to six months) should be given before the drug is considered a therapeutic failure. Those patients responding to therapy at six months often appear to lose their responsiveness months or years later, but the response can often be regained by reverting to an earlier more-frequent dosage schedule for a few weeks.

The most widely used dosage schedules are derived empirically from the protocol used by the British Empire Rheumatism Council in their landmark study carried out in the late 1950s and early 1960s. Little scientific evidence shows that major departures from this approach offer any real advantages, but minor departures for reasons of patient or physician convenience probably do not offer any significant disadvantages.

For simplicity only one protocol will be outlined here (Fig. 4-2), but minor variations are widely employed. The doses given are for adults; childhood doses are a matter of opinion, but probably average 0.5 mg/kg per injection. All injections are intramuscular. Baseline complete blood counts and urinalyses are obtained, and either GSTM or GSTG is given in test doses of first 10 mg and then a few days later 25 mg to be sure there is no hypersensitivity to the agent or its vehicle. Then a 50-mg injection is given once a week for about 20 weeks or to a total dose of 1 gm. Meanwhile toxicity monitoring requires frequent preinjection complete blood counts and urinalyses, preferably before each of the first 20. If no beneficial response is apparent at 1 gm, an additional four to six weeks of therapy might be elected. It is often difficult to persuade the patient to comply with this recommendation, and many clinicians will abandon the therapy as a failure at this point. Objective as well as subjective responses should be carefully evaluated before a decision is made. For this purpose detailed records of swollen and tender joints are especially helpful.

If evidence exists for a beneficial response at 20 weeks or 1 gm, the 50-mg injections may be given every two weeks for an additional three months. It is usually permissible to reduce the frequency of the laboratory monitoring at this time, since renal and hematologic toxicity are less likely after the first six months of treatment. At this point it might be elected to obtain the laboratory tests before every other injection. If improvement is continuing after three

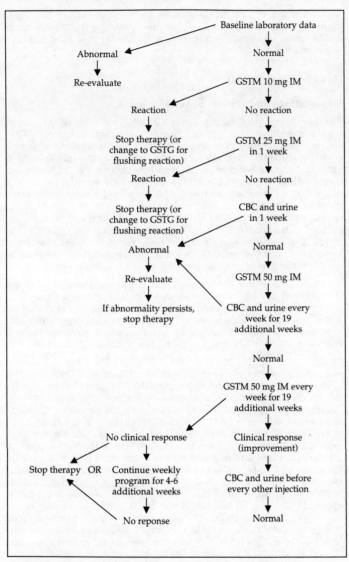

Fig. 4-2. Approach to parenteral gold therapy. (GSTM, gold sodium thiomalate; GSTG, gold sodium thioglucose.)

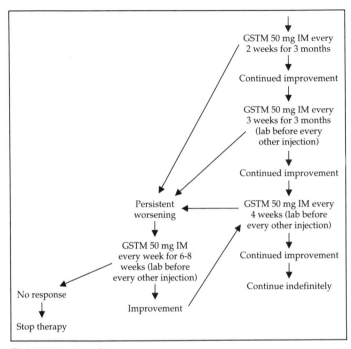

Fig. 4-2. (continued)

months of the biweekly schedule, the frequency of the 50-mg injections can be reduced to every three weeks for three additional months and then every four weeks if the improvement continues. Once a month is the usual maintenance schedule, and this program is continued as long as there is a satisfactory clinical response or indefinitely. At this time the therapy becomes relatively inexpensive and convenient to the patient, and it may be possible to withdraw anti-inflammatory therapies, further limiting the expense.

For patients who experience a persisting flare in disease activity during maintenance chrysotherapy, an apparent response can often be regained by increasing the frequency of the 50-mg injections for a few weeks. Several schedules have been recommended but none has been shown to be more effective than another. One approach would be to revert to a weekly schedule until improvement became apparent and then rapidly or gradually return to the every four-week program. It should be possible to recruit a satisfactory response in about half of these "secondary failures."

Clinical Aspects of Side Effects and Contraindications

Side effects reported from parenteral chrysotherapy are listed in Table 4-3. The vasomotor reaction consists of flushing, headache, syncope or near-syncope, nausea, and sweating. It occurs within a few minutes of a GSTM injection and is relatively common. It tends to recur with subsequent GSTM injections but is usually abolished

Table 4-3. Side effects of parenteral chrysotherapy

Postinjection reactions
    Vasomotor (flushing or "nitritoid")
    Arthralgias/myalgias (arthritis flare)
Mucocutaneous reactions
    Pruritus (often generalized)
    Dermatitis (often generalized)
    Stomatitis
    Alopecia
    Metallic taste
Renal complications
    Proteinuria
    Nephrotic syndrome
Hematopoietic complications
    Eosinophilia
    Leukopenia
    Thrombocytopenia
    Aplastic anemia
Rare or equivocal
    Diffuse pulmonary infiltrates ("gold lung")
    Enterocolitis
    Cholestatic jaundice
    Peripheral neuropathy

by changing to GSTG. What is perceived as a flare in the arthritis
occurring within a few hours of a GSTM injection is reported by
10–15% of patients receiving this agent. It also tends to recur with
GSTM injections and can usually be avoided by changing to GSTG.
The most common parenteral gold reactions are dermatitis and stomatitis. Rashes are reported by as many as 20% of patients receiving
parenteral chrysotherapy and are the most common side effect leading to its withdrawal. Of course, many of these rashes are not related
to the gold itself. Generalized pruritus is a typical prodrome, but
the skin lesion is polymorphous, usually precluding a precise dermatologic diagnosis. Unless the rash is severe, suggesting that permanent withdrawal of therapy would be prudent, it is reasonable
to withhold the injections until it clears and then cautiously restart
therapy with a low dose (10–25 mg) and slowly build back up to the
previous schedule. Stomatitis occurs in about 5% of patients receiving parenteral chrysotherapy and is more likely than skin symptoms
to result in permanently stopping the treatment, perhaps because
it is more likely to be due to the gold than are the rashes. Both
stomatitis and dermatitis tend to occur early in the course of gold
therapy, but they should be inquired about routinely before any
injection is given. Topical corticosteroids may benefit both the dermatitis and the stomatitis.

Significant proteinuria develops in about 1–3% of patients receiving
parenteral gold and also tends to occur early in the course of therapy.
A 1+ (30 mg) or greater protein on urine dipstick should lead to
withholding the injection, and if it persists at the time the next one
is due, a 24-hour urine should be collected to quantify protein excretion. If the protein excretion is significant (over 200–400 mg/24
hours), chrysotherapy should be permanently discontinued. Contin-

ued gold therapy in this case poses a significant risk for the nephrotic syndrome, which may also occur suddenly without a proteinuria prodrome being detected. Gold-induced nephrotic syndrome is usually reversible, but, of course, it should be prevented whenever possible. No specific therapy is available, though high-dose corticosteroid therapy has been thought to benefit some cases.

The most common hematologic abnormality in patients receiving gold is eosinophilia, which may be the forerunner of a serious problem; therefore, it is probably wise to withhold the injections until marked eosinophilia clears. Leukopenia or thrombocytopenia, presumably related to peripheral mechanisms, occurs in 1–3% of patients receiving parenteral gold, and the cytopenias tend to occur early in the course of therapy. RA itself may be a cause of the leukopenia, but the disease does not cause thrombocytopenia. If the platelet count or white blood cell count drops below normal during the course of chrysotherapy, and any doubt exists concerning the cause, the injections should be withheld. If the abnormality persists, in the absence of any other obvious cause, gold should be permanently discontinued. Severe degrees of leukopenia or thrombocytopenia have been treated with high-dose corticosteroids with reported successes, and gold chelation therapy has also been used; however, the cytopenias tend to slowly resolve without other therapy after the chrysotherapy is stopped. Gold does not cause an isolated anemia and need not be withdrawn for a fall in the red blood cell count.

The most dreaded complication of parenteral chrysotherapy is aplastic anemia, which may occur in 1 in 500–1000 treated patients. It may not be preventable with even the most careful of hematologic monitoring. Most reports have suggested a mortality in excess of 50%, but one recent series of 10 cases suggested a much more favorable prognosis. Therapies have included gold chelation, high-dose corticosteroids, androgens, bone marrow transplant, and antithymocyte globulin; the latter may be the most effective medical therapy.

The rapid development of symptomatic diffuse pulmonary infiltrates ("gold lung") is probably the best documented of the rare reactions. It is usually treated with high-dose corticosteroids. Although rare, patients should be aware of the reaction so they will report pulmonary symptoms at their onset. The appearance of cholestatic jaundice and symptoms of dysentery during gold therapy will usually require that it be permanently stopped. Neuropathy is more controversial since it may result from the RA itself; however, neuropathic symptoms should be carefully evaluated while the injections are being withheld.

Prevention of serious gold reactions is not always possible, but the more careful the laboratory monitoring the better. The blood count and urinalysis reports should be examined by a physician before the injection is given. In addition the physician or nurse should ask about pruritus, rashes, oral symptoms, and pulmonary symptoms before each shot. Although careful patient selection might help minimize the risk for reactions, a few absolute contraindications to chrysotherapy exist, the major one being a prior serious reaction to parenteral gold. Gold has been used without complication in patients with renal insufficiency, though it is probably wise to reduce the dose or frequency of injections. Certain pre-existing conditions could make toxicity monitoring difficult, e.g., proteinuria or leukopenia; however, chrysotherapy has been used safely in Felty's syndrome and may actually induce a remission in patients with that condition. Older patients do not appear to be at significant increased risk for side effects of chrysotherapy. Parenteral gold should not be given to pregnant women, and its use in nursing mothers is controversial.

Clinical Indications

GSTM and GSTG are indicated in "selected cases of active RA—both adult and juvenile type." In the juvenile RA syndromes, there are few controlled observations, but parenteral chrysotherapy is thought to be effective in the more serious polyarticular forms of the disease. Although there are no controlled studies, parenteral chrysotherapy has also been reported to be safe and effective in psoriatic arthritis, but it does not appear to benefit the other spondyloarthropathies. Not enough data exist to recommend these agents in any other rheumatic diseases, though they have been reported to benefit pemphigus.

Expense*

The cost of the drug to the patient will be about $10.00/50-mg injection. To this must be added the charges for giving the injection and the charges for the laboratory studies. An example is given in Table 4-4. Costs can be minimized by limiting the physicians' charges and by performing only the dipstick part of the urinalysis. Obviously the initial few months of therapy are quite expensive, but parenteral gold becomes one of the least expensive slow-acting therapies once the maintenance stage is reached.

Table 4-4. Estimated cost of parenteral chrysotherapy

Assume the following costs:	
Drug	$10
Injection charge	15
Blood count (with differential)	15
Urinalysis (dipstick)	8
Weeks 1–22 (lab every injection)	
10-mg test dose	$ 40
25-mg test dose	43
20–50-mg injections	960
	$1043
Weeks 23–35 (lab every other injection)	
Six 50-mg injections	$219
Weeks 36–48 (lab every other injection)	
Four 50-mg injections	$146
Total cost for loading period = $1408	
Cost/yr of maintenance (lab every other injection)	
Twelve 50-mg injections	$438

*All subsequent drug therapy laboratory and pharmacy expenses are estimates based on 1990 charges at one university hospital.

ORAL GOLD: AURANOFIN

Expectations and Dosage Schedules in RA

Auranofin has been widely used for over 10 years, and numerous controlled clinical trials clearly support its efficacy as a SAARD in RA. Although earlier studies suggested an efficacy approaching that of parenteral gold, more recent trials and clinical experience suggest a significantly lower beneficial response rate—perhaps about two-thirds that of the parenteral preparations. Preliminary studies suggest that auranofin might favorably affect the two-year outcome when used very early in the course of the disease, however. No response is expected before about three months of therapy, and at least six months are required before the drug can be considered a failure. More benefits might be expected if the drug is used early in the course of the disease.

The recommended adult dose is 6 mg/day in a single or divided daily dosage schedule. At six months the dose may be increased to 9 mg/ day for an additional three-month trial for those patients not responding to the lower dose, but this practice has not been adequately studied. Probably most American rheumatologists are willing to declare auranofin a failure after six months of 6 mg/day. For those patients responding at six months, the drug may be continued indefinitely. Later "secondary" failures are common and may respond to a few weeks to a few months of 9 mg/day, but, again, this practice has not been studied adequately. Recommended laboratory toxicity monitoring consists of a complete blood count and urinalysis once a month, continued as long as the patient takes the drug.

Clinical Aspects of Side Effects

Clearly auranofin has significantly less serious toxicity than do the parenteral gold compounds, and the early withdrawal rate because of all side effects is also lower than with parenteral gold. Withdrawal rates vary widely from study to study but are probably less than 10% in practice. Major auranofin side effects are listed in Table 4-5. By far the most common side effects are variations on the theme of loose stools, diarrhea, and lower abdominal discomfort. Taken together these symptoms occur in almost half of patients taking auranofin. In many cases the symptoms are mild and tolerable and

Table 4-5. Major auranofin side effects

Common
   Loose stools or diarrhea
   Abdominal discomfort
   Nausea

Less common than with parenteral gold
   Pruritus
   Rash
   Stomatitis

Much less common than with parenteral gold
   Proteinuria
   Leukopenia
   Thrombocytopenia

many others respond to symptomatic therapy; bismuth subsalicylate (Pepto-Bismol) has been shown to be especially effective in many of these cases. Nonetheless lower gastrointestinal complications are the most common side effects leading to auranofin withdrawal. Nausea is a frequent upper gastrointestinal complaint, but it often improves with time and continued therapy.

Rashes, with and without pruritus, were reported by about 25% of the patients taking auranofin in the premarketing studies, but skin reactions appear to be much less common in practice and only occasionally necessitate withdrawal of the drug. Likewise stomatitis seems to be equally uncommon in practice though it was reported by 13% of the patients in the premarketing trials. Clearly mucocutaneous reactions are less common with auranofin than with parenteral gold.

Proteinuria, thrombocytopenia, and leukopenia—the potentially serious reactions—were each reported in about 1% of the auranofin-treated patients in the premarketing trials, but they appear to be rare in the more recent studies and in clinical practice. Nevertheless, it would be prudent to follow the manufacturer's recommendation of a monthly complete blood count and urinalysis. These recommendations may be eased somewhat in the future. Since many patients taking auranofin are seen relatively infrequently by the physician, some mechanism must be established to ensure a reasonable compliance with the monthly laboratory tests.

It is uncertain whether a serious reaction to one form of gold (oral versus parenteral) implies a similar reaction to the other, but the nephrotic syndrome or serious hemocytopenias with one preparation do discourage the use of the other.

Clinical Indications and Contraindications

Auranofin is indicated only for active adult RA. A recent large international study of the drug in juvenile RA showed only marginal benefits though virtually no significant toxicity. No sufficient data exist to suggest that the drug might benefit other rheumatic conditions.

Should the drug be tried after parenteral gold has failed? This question cannot be answered on the basis of any scientific study; however, rheumatologists are probably not too enthusiastic about trying it under these circumstances. Patients frequently ask about changing parenteral to oral gold with expense and convenience in mind. The usual answer is that maintenance parenteral gold is more convenient and less expensive (and probably more effective) than the oral preparation.

The reverse situation—changing from oral to parenteral therapy— arises even more frequently, typically in patients who have failed to respond to auranofin. Again, few scientific data exist to support the practice, but it is done quite commonly with apparent benefits resulting. In that case, the number of weekly 50-mg injections required to induce a clinical response could be fewer than 20, and many clinicians will begin to reduce their frequency as soon as benefits become apparent, even if the cumulative parenteral dose is less than 1 g; however, it is still recommended that a total cumulative dose of 1 gm be given before the parenteral preparation is considered a failure.

No significant contraindications exist to the use of auranofin except prior serious toxicity and pregnancy. It has been well tolerated in patients with renal insufficiency.

Expense

At 6 mg/day, a month's supply of auranofin will cost the patient about $60. Considering that a complete blood count and urinalysis together cost about $23, the total cost for the month would be $83, and a year's therapy would cost almost $1000. Although this is less than the first year of parenteral gold therapy, the expense of auranofin does not diminish with time. Consequently after the first year, auranofin will cost over twice as much as maintenance parenteral gold (see Table 4-4).

D-Penicillamine

Because of pharmacologic actions likely irrelevant to its effects on RA, D-penicillamine has been used since the 1950s for the treatment of Wilson's disease and since the 1960s for cystinuria. In the 1950s it was found that D-penicillamine and other thiols could dissociate certain macroglobulins in vitro, leading to the observation that the drug resulted in a fall in RF titer when given to patients with RA. In the course of these experiments, improvement in the activity of the RA was noted in some patients, leading to the first controlled clinical trial of the drug in that disease in the early 1970s. Although the mechanism of action remains unknown, numerous controlled studies since have supported the original observation that D-penicillamine is an effective SAARD in RA, perhaps as effective as parenteral gold. Even though it is effective and has been approved and marketed for use in RA for about 10 years, the toxicity of the drug and its very gradual onset of action limit the current enthusiasm for its use.

D-penicillamine is an oral drug, available in 125-mg and 250-mg capsules as Cuprimine, and in 250-mg scored tablets as Depen. The preparations may be used interchangeably.

BASIC PHARMACOLOGY

General Properties

D-penicillamine (β, β-dimethylcysteine), an analog of the natural amino acid, D-cysteine, was isolated as an hydrolysis product of penicillin (structure, Fig. 4-3). It is a water-soluble, active sulfhydryl reagent capable of chelating metals, including gold, zinc, copper, mercury, and lead, and of participating in sulfhydryl-disulfide exchange reactions. The former is the mechanism that accounts for the effectiveness of penicillamine in lowering copper levels in Wilson's disease, as well as its utility in mobilizing other metals; the latter is the mechanism by which penicillamine exchanges with one of the two cysteines of the disulfide compound cystine. Cystine is relatively water insoluble and, in cystinuria, can result in renal stones/precipitation. The exchange compound, penicillamine-cysteine, is more soluble. Actions of penicillamine that may relate to its efficacy in RA are briefly reviewed in the following sections.

Mechanisms of Action

Sulfhydryl-Disulfide Exchange

As mentioned in the previous section on gold compounds, free sulfhydryl availability, even associated with plasma albumin, is decreased in RA and may be related to elevated immunoglobulins and immune complex formation involving formation of disulfide bonds. D-penicillamine exchange in such disulfide bonds would simultaneously reduce macromolecular weights and increase sulfhydryl availability. One consequence could include dissociation of RF, the original rationale for use of penicillamine in RA. In patients treated with penicillamine, an increase occurs in intracellular levels of (reduced) glutathione, an agent whose availability can modulate activity of peroxidases and also superoxide production (Fig. 4-3).

Interference with cross-link formation in collagen through formation of penicillamine complexes has been suggested. Presumably this would increase soluble collagen and decrease more antigenic, higher weight forms; however, whether all types of collagen are favorably influenced is unclear.

Dismutation of Superoxide

Penicillamine's ability to complex with copper also may be involved in its antirheumatic effects: Copper-penicillamine accelerates the dismutation of superoxide, i.e., it acts analogously to the enzyme superoxide dismutase. Superoxide anion (O_2^{-}) released by activated neutrophils and monocytes/macrophages is a proposed mediator of chronic inflammation. Superoxide's effects may include alteration of structures/macromolecules leading to destruction or to increased antigenicity, or to both. Importantly, superoxide dismutase, which accelerates conversion of superoxide to less toxic products (Fig. 4-3), is an intracellular enzyme and essentially absent from synovial fluid. Penicillamine gains access to synovial fluid and indeed is stabilized by the acidic environment created by ongoing inflammatory processes in the joint space. Dismutation of superoxide is thus a probable local anti-inflammatory mechanism of penicillamine. Additional therapeutic benefit may also come from superoxide dismutation.

Immunosuppression

A product of superoxide dismutation is hydrogen peroxide (H_2O_2). Penicillamine, in the presence of copper and a source of superoxide, through the product H_2O_2, reportedly inhibits antigen-induced T-lymphocyte proliferation without effect on B-lymphocyte proliferation. T-helper subpopulations appear most sensitive. Penicillamine-treated lymphocytes, including those obtained from patients, reportedly elicit less collagenase secretion from cultured synovial cells, suggesting decreased mediator release. In contrast to other antirheumatic drugs, penicillamine has little effect on monocytes. It has

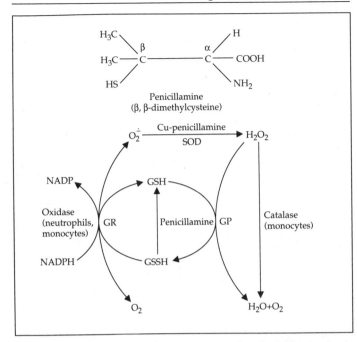

Fig. 4-3. Some mechanisms of penicillamine action. Penicillamine (top) can affect levels of reduced glutathione (GSH), and thus decrease lipid peroxidation reactions. Cu-penicillamine can promote the dismutation of superoxide ($O_2^{\cdot}$) to H_2O_2, which may be immunosuppressant (inhibition of T-lymphocyte proliferation). Catalase released from monocytes may remove H_2O_2 and limit its effect. (SOD, superoxide dismutase; GR, glutathione reductase; GP, glutathione peroxidase.)

been suggested that, because of their high content of catalase (which breaks down H_2O_2), monocytes can influence the immunosuppressant effects of penicillamine.

Pyridoxal phosphate (vitamin B_6) complexes with penicillamine. It has been suggested that removal of this important enzyme cofactor contributes to immunosuppression. This mechanism, even if involved, would be insufficient alone to account for the drug's effects, however.

Mechanisms of Side Effects and Toxicity

Side effects are common with penicillamine therapy and may be increased in individuals with decreased sulfoxidation conjugation capacity, i.e., decreased ability to biotransform penicillamine. It also has been suggested that, as for gold, certain haplotypes, possibly HLA-DR3, predispose to side effect occurrence.

Adverse changes in renal function, specifically immune complex nephritis with proteinuria, can occur in up to a third of treated patients. This would suggest, as for gold, the possibility that some sulfhydryl-disulfide exchanges may result in altered macromolecular structures against which an immune response is mounted. In support of this, occasional association of penicillamine therapy with development of a lupus-like syndrome or other autoimmune-type responses has been noted.

Hematologic effects of penicillamine, including thrombocytopenia, leukopenia, and even aplastic anemia, occur via unknown mechanisms. The cytotoxic mechanisms that are proposed to occur for gold, and that may again involve sulfhydryl-disulfide exchanges and functional impairment of normal processes, may or may not apply.

The mechanism for another common side effect of penicillamine, namely skin rashes, is unknown. In theory, skin rashes could result from hypersensitivity, consistent with immune complex renal injury and autoimmune syndrome occurrence. Documentation to support this premise is lacking, however.

EXPECTATIONS AND DOSAGE SCHEDULES IN RA

The efficacy of D-penicillamine depends on its daily dosage over a period of at least two to three months. A minimum effective dose is 500 mg/day, and about 750 mg/day is required to produce a beneficial response rate similar to that of parenteral gold; therefore, D-penicillamine is one of the more effective SAARDs, but it is also one of the more toxic. At the doses required to produce an effect similar to that of parenteral gold, the withdrawal rate due to side effects may be as high as 40% in the first year or so of therapy. At least two months of an effective dose are required before benefits become apparent, and the response may be delayed as long as four to six months. Consequently D-penicillamine can be a very slow-acting agent.

It is generally thought that toxicity can be minimized by using the drug in a "go low—go slow" fashion allowing at least two and preferably three months between dosage increments, which could be either 125 mg or 250 mg depending on the patient's tolerance. Because of toxicity it is preferable not to exceed a dose of 750 mg/day, but some patients will require 1000 mg/day in order to achieve a satisfactory response. It is therefore apparent that a year or longer could be required for drug failure to become apparent, and most physicians and patients are not willing to adhere to an unrewarding program over this long a period. A more acceptable (but more risky) approach might be to give 250 mg/day for a month or so as a test dose and then increase to 500 mg/day for three months and then to 750 mg/day if no response is apparent; if no beneficial effects occur after three months of 750 mg/day, the drug might be considered a failure. This more rapid schedule might increase the risk of side effects and will fail to identify a few potential responders, but it might also retain a few disenchanted patients who would otherwise have dropped out of the program. Once an effective dose is identified, it is continued indefinitely. Late failures may respond to further dose increments if they can be tolerated, but the daily dose should not exceed 1000 mg. D-penicillamine should always be taken in the postabsorptive state with no other drugs taken simultaneously.

Meanwhile toxicity monitoring should consist of a complete blood count and urinalysis every two weeks for the first few months of therapy and then every three to four weeks depending on the final dose. At least monthly laboratory tests are continued as long as the patient continues the drug.

CLINICAL ASPECTS OF SIDE EFFECTS

The incidence of various side effects due to D-penicillamine is difficult to estimate since they appear to be dose-dependent. The side effects tend to cluster in the first year or so of therapy with any given dose and become less likely as therapy proceeds unless the dose is increased. Reports suggest that side effects are more common in patients with RA than in patients with Wilson's disease and cystinuria, but this may be simply because the drug is more often used in RA. Established D-penicillamine side effects are listed in Table 4-6.

Hypogeusia, or loss of taste, is quite common and often improves even if the therapy is continued. Early pruritus and rashes are often trivial and may respond to symptomatic therapy while the D-penicillamine is continued; however, rashes occurring later in the course of therapy are often more serious and frequently require that the drug be stopped. Stomatitis may also vary from mild to severe but is less of a problem with D-penicillamine than with parenteral chrysotherapy. Persisting nausea, often with anorexia, is a common reason for stopping therapy. Occasionally these symptoms can be made more tolerable by giving the drug at bedtime.

Thrombocytopenia and leukopenia, presumably due to peripheral mechanisms, are more common with D-penicillamine than with parenteral gold, but aplastic anemia may be less common. Any significant drop below normal in white blood cell or platelet count should result in drug withdrawal. It is sometimes possible to reinstitute

Table 4-6. Established D-penicillamine side effects

Common and usually not serious
    Hypogeusia
    Dermatitis
    Stomatitis
    Nausea
    Anorexia
Relatively common and potentially serious
    Thrombocytopenia
    Leukopenia
    Proteinuria/nephrotic syndrome
Uncommon and potentially serious
    Aplastic anemia
    Induction of autoimmune disease
        Myasthenia gravis
        Pemphigus
        Systemic lupus erythematosus
        Goodpasture's syndrome
        Polymyositis
        Sjögren's syndrome (?)

therapy at a lower dose after the count returns to normal, but the lower dose may not be effective enough to justify continuing it. Proteinuria and the nephrotic syndrome are also more common with D-penicillamine than with parenteral gold. Significant proteinuria, documented by a 24-hour urine measurement, should result in at least temporary drug withdrawal. It is sometimes possible to restart D-penicillamine after the proteinuria clears, but, again, the lower dose may not be effective.

The most curious and confounding side effects of D-penicillamine are the autoimmune disorders that it has been reported to induce. Individually these are rare, some representing only a few case reports, but they are potentially serious. Any clinical suggestion of any one of the disorders listed in Table 4-6 should result in D-penicillamine withdrawal. If the diagnosis can be documented, the drug should not be restarted.

CLINICAL INDICATIONS AND CONTRAINDICATIONS

Besides Wilson's disease and cystinuria, D-penicillamine is indicated only for active, severe RA. It has also been shown to be effective in polyarticular juvenile RA though the childhood dose schedule has not been well established. Several observations suggest that the drug might be particularly useful in certain extra-articular manifestations of RA, including vasculitis, interstitial lung disease, Felty's syndrome, and amyloidosis. A few uncontrolled observations suggest that psoriatic arthritis might benefit from D-penicillamine therapy. Preliminary studies also suggest a role in systemic sclerosis; in doses similar to those recommended for RA, some improvement in the skin and pulmonary manifestations have been noted.

D-penicillamine may be effective and well tolerated in patients with RA who have demonstrated no response or toxicity to other slow-acting agents, especially parenteral gold.

The only contraindications to the drug are prior serious toxicity to it and pregnancy. Allergy to penicillin does not predict an untoward reaction to D-penicillamine. It has been used safely in patients with renal insufficiency, but at much lower doses than those recommended previously.

EXPENSE

The expense of D-penicillamine therapy depends on the dose. Thirty 250-mg capsules or tablets will cost the patient about $30. Assuming a "go low—go slow" approach with 250-mg dose increments every two months, initial laboratory monitoring every two weeks, and a final dose of 750 mg/day, the first six months of therapy would cost $636 ($360 for the drug and $276 for the laboratory tests). If laboratory testing were decreased to every three weeks for the second six months, the cost would be $724 ($540 for the drug and $184 for the laboratory). With monthly laboratory monitoring after the first year and a regular dose of 750 mg/day, the annual cost would be $1356 ($1080 for the drug and $276 for the laboratory). Consequently maintenance D-penicillamine is significantly more expensive than maintenance parenteral chrysotherapy.

Azathioprine

Azathioprine is a prodrug that is metabolized to its active form 6-mercaptopurine (6MP). It was designed in the 1960s specifically to be a well-tolerated agent for the prevention of renal transplant rejection. Its immunosuppressive properties naturally lead to trials in patients with presumed autoimmune diseases, particularly RA, and controlled studies began to appear in the late 1960s and early 1970s. Since then a number of controlled clinical trials have clearly documented its efficacy as a slow-acting agent in that disease, with a response rate similar to that of parenteral gold and D-penicillamine. It has been approved by the FDA for use in RA for about 10 years.

Parenteral azathioprine has rarely been used in any of the autoimmune diseases, so only the oral preparation will be discussed here. It is only available as Imuran in 50-mg scored tablets. Emphasizing its approved use in RA, the drug has been marketed as ImuRAn.

BASIC PHARMACOLOGY

General Properties and Mechanisms

The properties and activities of 6MP and azathioprine, which is converted in vivo to 6MP, are essentially identical. Azathioprine has better oral absorption characteristics, which, combined with its longer time action, accounts for its use in preference to 6MP. Discussion of these compounds will therefore proceed with usual reference to azathioprine, with the understanding that the data apply equally to 6MP, except where noted. For reference, the structures and some conversions of azathioprine and 6MP are shown in Fig. 4-4.

Azathioprine is a substituted analog of the naturally occurring purine, guanine. Azathioprine is inactive, i.e., it is a prodrug, and must be converted to 6MP, an analog of hypoxanthine, for the majority of its activity. The necessity for conversion and the time required for it result in a total half-life of about five hours, considerably longer than that of 6MP ($\approx$ one hour). Some conversion to thioguanine (6TG), another analog with actions similar to 6MP, has also been suggested. Nonenzymatic conversion of azathioprine to 6MP, by reaction with sulfhydryl compounds such as glutathione, has been suggested; however, enzymatic conversion also takes place in the liver. Importantly, compromised liver function apparently limits or even prevents the immunosuppressant actions of azathioprine in humans.

Azathioprine belongs to the general class of drugs known as **antimetabolites**, an indication of its general mechanism of action. It was originally proposed that purine analogs were simply incorporated as "false bases" into DNA and thus interfered with DNA replication, and so forth. Although substitution may occur, additional, and important, mechanisms have been identified for the reduction in DNA replication induced by azathioprine.

Azathioprine, after conversion to 6MP, which is a substrate for the purine salvage pathway enzyme HGPRT (hypoxanthine-guanine

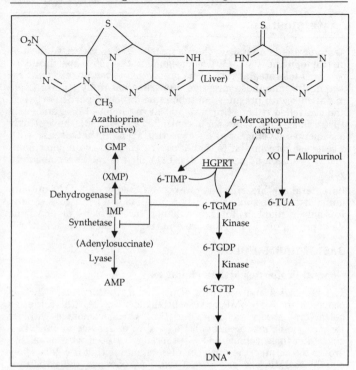

Fig. 4-4. Biotransformations of azathioprine to active species. Following formation of 6-mercaptopurine (6MP), the 6MP is further converted to 6-thioIMP (6-TIMP) (main) and to 6-thioGMP (6-GDP, GTP) (6-TGMP) (minor), both of which inhibit further activity of the hypoxanthine-guanine phosphoribosyl transferase (HGPRT) salvage pathway and also enzymes that convert inosine monophosphate (IMP) to adenosine monophosphate (AMP) and guanosine monophosphate (diphosphate, triphosphate) (GMP). 6-TGMP can also be additionally phosphated and incorporated into DNA (* modified). Conversion to inactive 6-thiouric acid (6-TUA) can be blocked by allopurinol. (—, inhibits; XMP, xanthosine monophosphate; XO, xanthine oxidase.)

phosphoribosyl transferase), is converted to 6TIMP (6-**t**hio-**i**nosine 5'-**m**ono**p**hosphate). Since 6TIMP is a poor substrate for the enzyme (guanylate kinase) that converts native IMP to its nucleotide **d**i**p**hosphate, only a very small fraction is converted to 6TIDP, and 6TIMP accumulates. Accumulation of 6TIMP acts to prevent formation of nucleotides, in part by feedback inhibition of HGPRT, but also by inhibiting enzymes involved in the conversion of IMP to AMP and GMP (Fig. 4-4, bottom) as well as in de novo purine biosynthesis. As mentioned before, azathioprine (6MP) is also converted to 6TG, another substrate for HGPRT, resulting in formation of 6TGMP (6-**t**hio-**g**uanosine **m**ono**p**hosphate). Like 6TIMP, 6TGMP inhibits de novo purine biosynthesis. It should be noted that in contrast to 6TIMP, 6TGMP is an effective substrate for guanylate kinase and

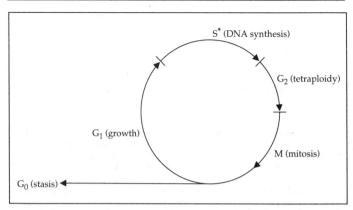

Fig. 4-5. Standard cell growth cycle showing phases. S*-phase drugs discussed under SAARDs include azathioprine (6-mercaptopurine) and methotrexate. Nonphase specific (cycle-specific) drugs include cyclophosphamide and chlorambucil.

is thus further converted to 6TGDP and 6TGTP. The latter can be incorporated into DNA. Although the incidence of HGPRT deficiency is low, it is worth noting that individuals with such a deficiency would be resistant to effects of azathioprine.

In addition to the aforementioned conversions, 6MP is converted by xanthine oxidase to an inactive metabolite, 6-thiouric acid. The drug allopurinol (see Chapter 5 for details) was developed to inhibit this conversion and prolong the duration and intensity of action of 6MP. Addition of allopurinol to a therapeutic regimen that includes azathioprine or 6MP may require significant decreases (up to 75%) in usual doses to avoid unwanted effects.

Azathioprine (6MP) is a phase-specific drug, i.e., it affects cells in a particular state of growth, the S-phase, more so than at other stages (Figure 4-5). Although effects on S-phase are primary, azathioprine can also affect RNA and protein synthesis in growth phases G_1 and G_2, although higher doses may be required. Since G_1 precedes S-phase, which is much more sensitive to drug effects, high drug level effects at G_1 can actually prevent entry into S-phase and thus limit the degree of cytotoxicity. Thus, azathioprine (6MP) is sometimes referred to as an S-phase specific, self-limited (class 2) drug.

Although the effects of azathioprine are anticipated to be widespread, the drug targets proliferating cells and has a differing degree of effect in proportion to the degree of proliferative activity. Also, certain subpopulations of cells appear to be more sensitive than others, which may be of significance in immunomodulatory effects.

Immunomodulatory Mechanisms

Azathioprine has been noted to cause a peripheral lymphopenia after several months of administration to RA patients. The reduction includes both B- and T-lymphocytes, and only rarely has a differential effect in the latter population been reported (greater reduction in T-helper). In contrast, patients given larger amounts of azathioprine to suppress graft rejection, for example, have clear reductions in T-helpers. Spleen and thymus DNA and RNA content are significantly reduced in animals treated with immunosuppressant (in contrast to cytotoxic) doses of azathioprine in vivo, and decreases in immunoglobulin levels, due to reduced synthesis rate, are observed.

B-lymphocyte function appears to be modified by azathioprine. Antibody production is reduced, and this may be more or less restricted to secondary IgG production. The latter has been stated to indicate a site of effect at terminal B-cell differentiation. Since T-suppressor function is very sensitive to azathioprine, more so than B-cells in general, low doses of azathioprine may actually accentuate B-antibody responses.

Azathioprine inhibits responses of mixed lymphocyte populations (T- and B-proliferation in the presence of specific antigen) at very low doses, but only if included at initiation. The inhibitory effect of azathioprine is not reversed by inclusion of IL-2, suggesting that mediator release by stimulated T-helpers is not involved. One suggestion is that antigen recognition is somehow impaired. It has been suggested that surface receptor expression may be altered; this is supported, in part, by decreased T-rosetting of sheep erythrocytes subsequent to azathioprine therapy, but the relationship of this to antigen recognition is not clear. During in vivo use of azathioprine, inhibition of mixed lymphocyte responses has not been observed.

The cells that show the greatest inhibition by azathioprine are so-called NK (natural killer) cells, although K (killer) cells are also inhibited. K cells participate in antibody-dependent responses, whereas NK cells do not require antibody for subsequent response. Since specific roles for these cells in RA have not been documented, it is difficult to indicate what role their inhibition by azathioprine plays in the drug's overall therapeutic efficacy. The mechanism of azathioprine reduction in NK and K activity involves, in part, reductions in their populations.

Special Features and Mechanisms of Side Effects

A useful "side effect" of azathioprine **may** be an anti-inflammatory effect: 6MP has been observed to be significantly anti-inflammatory. One proposed mechanism (for 6MP) involves inhibition of monocyte chemotaxis. Further documentation of the effect and investigation of mechanism(s) are required, however.

The unwanted side effects of azathioprine therapy include bone marrow suppression, expressed as leukopenia or thrombocytopenia, or both. Its parent compound, 6MP, can produce severe hepatic toxicity (up to 30% of treated patients develop cholestatic jaundice), but this is usually in antineoplastic doses. Lower 6MP doses produce less toxicity. Azathioprine hepatotoxicity is significantly less than that of 6MP, possibly reflecting both lower usual doses and the relatively slow release of 6MP from the prodrug. Gastrointestinal toxicity (nausea, vomiting) is likewise seen but is less than with 6MP. The production of bone marrow suppression, hepatic damage, and gastrointestinal effects probably occurs via the biochemical mechanisms already described.

The degree of conversion of azathioprine to 6TGMP may influence the degree of toxicity seen. Neutropenic patients have considerably higher erythrocyte 6-TGMP than do non-neutropenic patients. Folic acid somehow influences the conversion of azathioprine (6MP) to 6TGMP: Administration of excess folic acid eliminates an otherwise linear relationship between 6MP administered and 6TGMP formed. Since it was not reported that folic acid eliminates desirable effects, this suggests that folic acid might be used to counter development of toxicity. Currently this is an intriguing, but totally undocumented premise.

Two additional potential side effects of azathioprine are worthy of mention: increased risk of infection and increased risk of neoplastic disease. Increased risk of infection is a direct result of immunosuppression and extends to almost any invading organism, even those that are not usually pathogenic. Increased risk of tumor is also a result primarily or only of immunosuppression, i.e., decreased immune surveillance, since low doses of azathioprine are not mutagenic. Tumor development risk is apparently quite real for doses of azathioprine used in energetic immunosuppression, e.g., in suppression of transplant rejection. The risk for doses used in RA is uncertain.

EXPECTATIONS AND DOSAGE SCHEDULES IN RA

Although there is some evidence that azathioprine may be effective in RA in doses of about 1 mg/kg/day ($<$ 100 mg/day), this evidence is not widely accepted and the drug is usually given in an initial dose of 100 mg/day. At this or higher doses, azathioprine is as effective as parenteral gold and D-penicillamine, usually with less reported toxicity and lower drop-out rates because of side effects. It takes at least 8, and as many as 12, weeks to judge the effectiveness of a given dose, and much of the toxicity is dose related; therefore, as with D-penicillamine, a "go-slow" approach to dose adjustments is indicated.

If no clinical response is apparent three months after starting 100 mg/day, the dose may be increased to 125 mg/day for an additional three months and then to 150 mg/day for three more months if no response is apparent at 125 mg/day. Even though the manufacturers recommend 2.5 mg/kg/day (about 175 mg) as the maximum dose, many clinicians prefer not to exceed 150 mg/day. Since the approach outlined here requires at least nine months to select out nonresponders, it is sometimes accelerated by going from 100 mg/day directly to 150 mg/day after three months. Some late or "secondary" drug failures may respond to further dose increments if they can be tolerated. For those responding to a given dosage schedule, it may be continued indefinitely or attempts may be made later to gradually reduce it in order to be certain that the lowest effective dose has been determined.

Meanwhile laboratory toxicity monitoring consists of a complete blood count every three to four weeks, depending on the dose of azathioprine, and periodic (perhaps every three months) tests for hepatotoxicity are also recommended.

The schedules and expectations detailed previously apply directly only to the use of azathioprine in RA. It is much less certain how to use the drug and what to expect of it when it is given to patients with systemic lupus erythematosus (SLE), polymyositis, Reiter's syndrome, and other rheumatic diseases in which it has been used. None of these represent FDA-approved indications.

CLINICAL ASPECTS OF SIDE EFFECTS.

As with D-penicillamine, azathioprine side effects tend to be dose-dependent, making generalizations concerning their frequency difficult; however, it is clear from the comparative studies that azathioprine is associated with less apparent toxicity than parenteral gold and D-penicillamine. Azathioprine should be used in much lower doses with extreme caution or not at all in patients taking allopurinol, which markedly delays its metabolism.

Nausea and vomiting are common minor side effects and are reported by about 10% of the patients taking the drug. These symptoms can often be minimized by giving the drug after meals or in divided doses. Significant hepatotoxicity occurs in less than 1% of RA patients receiving the drug, and tests for this reaction should be done about every three months.

Leukopenia occurring early in the course of therapy with low doses of azathioprine has been reported and is thought to be a hypersensitivity reaction. Otherwise leukopenia or thrombocytopenia reflects bone marrow suppression and is generally dose-dependent. About 5% of patients with RA receiving azathioprine will be found to have a hemocytopenia; the drug should be withheld until recovery is complete and then cautiously restarted in a lower dose. Life-threatening degrees of leukopenia or thrombocytopenia occur rarely. Although macrocytosis is rather common with azathioprine, macrocytic anemias are not.

In doses used for RA, it is likely that azathioprine directly predisposes only to herpetic infections, but, of course, severe degrees of neutropenia related to the drug may result in others that are more life threatening.

The most dreaded complication of azathioprine therapy in RA may not, in fact, exist. It is relatively clear that the drug is associated with an increased risk of malignancy, especially lymphoma, when it is used in renal transplant recipients. It is not at all clear that this experience can be transposed to the use of azathioprine in RA. Studies adequate to define the risk have not been done, and those that are published have yielded conflicting results. The uncertain nature of this issue has cast a pall over the use of the drug in RA, one that will not be lifted until the issue is finally settled. The question of oncogenicity has to be raised when the drug is discussed with patients who are prospective recipients; very often it will be their sole reason for rejecting it.

CLINICAL INDICATIONS AND CONTRAINDICATIONS

Azathioprine is FDA approved only for renal homotransplantation and adult severe active RA, but it is widely used for a variety of other diseases. It is usually not the first slow-acting agent chosen for RA, and prior experiences with other slow-acting drugs do not predict similar experiences with azathioprine.

Among the rheumatic diseases, in addition to RA, azathioprine has probably been most often used in SLE. The published experiences, using doses similar to those used in RA, suggest that azathioprine may exert a "steroid-sparing" effect in patients with active disease; that is, it may allow for a gradual reduction in corticosteroid dose that would not otherwise have been possible. Controlled studies in the more severe forms of lupus nephritis have yielded conflicting results, and other immunosuppressive approaches are more fashionable now (see Cyclophosphamide). A number of published experiences have suggested that azathioprine therapy of active SLE during pregnancy might result in a better maternal and fetal outcome, but it is generally recommended that the drug not be used during pregnancy. Presently the role of azathioprine in SLE is very uncertain and it is best regarded as experimental in that context.

One small controlled study suggested marginal and delayed benefits from azathioprine in patients with polymyositis. It has been used in Reiter's syndrome with a few documented successes. Beyond the rheumatic diseases, azathioprine does seem to benefit autoimmune chronic active hepatitis. Its role in other autoimmune disorders is too uncertain to deserve further comment here.

Azathioprine is contraindicated in patients with a prior serious reaction to it, in pregnant RA patients, and in patients with a known malignancy. It should be used in low doses and with extra caution in patients taking allopurinol and in patients with renal insufficiency. A prior malignancy considered cured or arrested is a relative contraindication, as in liver disease.

EXPENSE

Laboratory monitoring usually consists of a monthly complete blood count ($15) and a liver profile ($23) every three months. At 100 mg/day, the drug will cost the patient about $60/month. Consequently the first six months of therapy can be expected to cost about $609 if the dose is increased from 100 to 150 mg/day at three months ($159 for laboratory and $450 for the drug). Maintenance therapy at 150 mg/day would cost $1352 annually ($272 for laboratory and $1080 for the drug), which is almost identical to the annual cost of D-penicillamine therapy.

Antimalarials

Among the currently available antimalarial drugs, only quinacrine and certain quinoline derivatives have demonstrated antirheumatic effects, and, of these, only chloroquine and hydroxychloroquine

(HCQ) are widely used for this purpose. In this country most rheumatologists use only HCQ since it is thought to be less toxic than chloroquine.

The beneficial effects of quinine on lupus erythematosus were first reported in 1894. During the first half of this century, a number of derivatives became available and quinacrine was reported to benefit lupus in 1940. In the early 1950s, it was suggested that other antimalarials might be useful first in the arthritis of SLE and then in RA. Later in the 1950s, chloroquine was reported to benefit the majority of patients with RA, and controlled studies of both HCQ and chloroquine in RA were done in the latter 1950s and early 1960s. Since then, additional controlled trials, mostly involving chloroquine, have supported the efficacy of these drugs as slow-acting agents in RA. For reasons that are not entirely clear, these drugs do not appear to be as effective in practice as they were in the controlled trials; nonetheless, they qualify as legitimate slow-acting drugs in RA and are probably even more effective in discoid lupus erythematosus and certain other manifestations of SLE.

HCQ is available in 200-mg tablets as Plaquenil, and chloroquine is available in 250-mg and 500-mg tablets generically and as Aralen. The emphasis in this discussion will be on HCQ, since it is the one most widely used in this country and has been thought to be as effective as chloroquine.

BASIC PHARMACOLOGY

General Properties

The two antimalarial compounds to be discussed in this section are chloroquine and hydroxychloroquine. Since the actions of these compounds are identical, no distinction will be made between them, i.e., actions will be referenced to HCQ, consistent with the clinical applications section, but apply equally to chloroquine. For reference, the structures of chloroquine and HCQ are shown in Fig. 4-6.

The absorption of HCQ after oral administration is essentially complete. The drug is plasma bound ($< 60\%$; albumin, α_1-acid glycoprotein) but distributes widely but, due to extensive tissue binding and ion trapping, accumulates to impressive degrees in the lung, kidney, spleen, liver, melanin-containing tissues, and also leukocytes. The levels of drug found in tissues can be several hundred times that in plasma. For example, therapeutic levels in plasma are in the micromolar (μM; 1×10^{-6}M) range, whereas simultaneous levels in liver and leukocytes are 300–500 μM ($3–5 \times 10^{-4}$M) and in red cells only 0.1 μM. The pharmacokinetics of chloroquine are the subject of an excellent recent review (see Titus, Bibliography).

Biotransformation occurs primarily in the liver (de-ethylation), and both the parent drug and its metabolites are renally excreted. Because of the effect of extensive tissue binding on apparent elimination kinetics, dose-dependent elimination was thought to occur; however, this is probably not the case. The elimination kinetics of HCQ are indeed complex, with a main half-life of six to seven days and a very slow component with a half-life of about a month for a daily oral dose regimen.

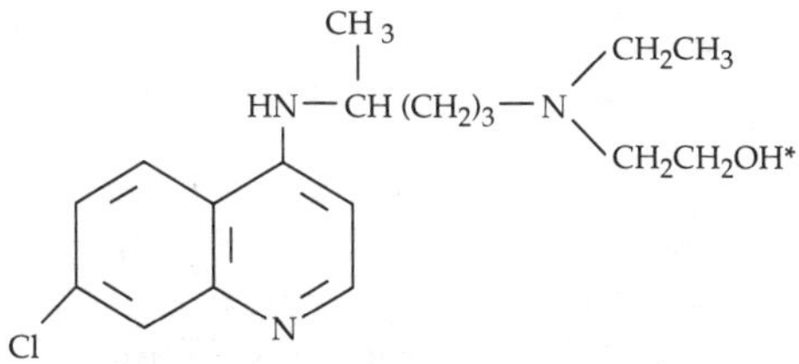

Hydroxychloroquine (HCQ)

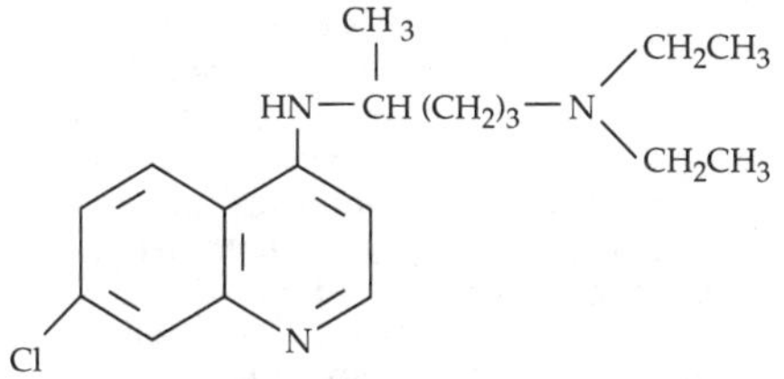

Chloroquine (CQ)

Fig. 4-6. Structures of antimalarials used in the therapy of rheumatoid arthritis. Hydroxychloroquine (HCQ) differs from chloroquine (CQ) only by an -OH(*) on the ethyl group attached to the terminal nitrogen. The two compounds are marketed in different salt forms, however (HCQ, sulfate; CQ, phosphate).

Mechanisms of Action

General Mechanisms

Several potential mechanisms may be involved in the beneficial effects of HCQ in RA. The degree of contribution to total effect made by any one of them is difficult to assess, although on a plasma concentration basis, they may be differentiated.

As mentioned before, HCQ accumulates in tissues. The accumulation results from both binding and ion trapping. The former reflects intercalation in DNA, binding to macromolecules, such as melanin, and binding to phospholipids. Ion trapping results from the chemical nature of HCQ and the prevailing pH in subcellular structures, e.g., lysosomes and endosomes. Like most drugs, HCQ exists in both ionized and unionized forms at physiologic pH. The unionized or lipophilic form can diffuse through membranes; the ionized form cannot. Initial movement of HCQ into cells and subcellular structures is thus accomplished by the freely permeant, unionized species. The pH inside lysosomes and endosomes, however, is low, and once inside these structures HCQ is almost completely protonated (ionized) and no longer able to diffuse through membranes; this process is referred to as **ion trapping**.

Many of the enzymes and other functions of the lysosomes and endosomes require low pH; the buffering effect, i.e., increased pH, caused by HCQ accumulation can inhibit pH-dependent, and other, processes. Importantly, at plasma concentrations achieved during antimalarial therapy, alkalinization of macrophage (monocyte) vesicles has been demonstrated, with the potential consequences described below.

The functions of endosomes and lysosomes are quite different. Briefly, one aspect of endosome function concerns recycling of cell surface receptors. Ligand-receptor complexes and some unoccupied receptors are internalized through vesicles that form from specialized membrane invaginations ("coated pits"). The latter vesicles fuse with endosomes, where either the ligand dissociates and is transferred to lysosomes where it is enzymatically destroyed, with the receptor then recycled to the cell surface, or the entire ligand-receptor complex is transferred and destroyed. In the latter case, new receptors are synthesized to replace the old. For those ligand-receptor complexes that usually dissociate, the dissociation is pH-dependent: pH 7 stabilizes most complexes; pH less than or equal to 5 favors dissociation. Thus, HCQ, by increasing endosomal pH, can interfere with receptor recycling and lead to decreases in numbers of receptors on the cell surface. In addition, new or recycled receptors are returned to the cell surface by exocytosis, another process limited by HCQ and possibly also by pH changes.

The functions of lysosomes are more familiar and therefore will not be described in detail. Lysosomal enzymes (acid hydrolases) are degradative and generally localized within the structure. Increased pH decreases the effectiveness of most lysosomal enzymes. Moreover, lysosomal release can occur during stimulation of some cells, e.g., neutrophils. Inhibition of vesicle fusion (exocytosis) by HCQ may thus also reduce lysosomal enzyme release from stimulated cells.

Immunomodulatory Mechanisms

The effects described previously can contribute to the overall effects of HCQ in RA; however, additional effects have been observed that are probably even more directly involved. Some of these relate to the decreased immunoglobulin and RF levels that are observed during HCQ therapy.

Direct effects on secretion of immunoglobulins occur only at very high HCQ levels and are therefore not considered to be a primary mechanism for HCQ. Indirect effects are probable, however. Inhibition of IL-1 release from monocytes/macrophages does occur in response to HCQ. Interference with this early signal to T-lymphocytes would also reduce T-helper elaboration of growth factor (IL-2) and thus decrease B-lymphocyte populations and immunoglobulin production. Since IL-2 elicits release of a sequence of other cytokines (see Chapter 3 for additional details) and indirectly acute phase proteins, HCQ's effect on IL-1 has potential for widespread beneficial consequences. Inhibition of IL-1 is also consistent with the observed anti-inflammatory activity of HCQ.

Macrophage processing and presentation of antigens involve both endocytosis and lysosomal enzyme activity, two processes interfered with by HCQ as described previously. HCQ can apparently interfere with appropriate codisplay of Ia (major histocompatibility complex class II) antigens during antigen processing and presentation. Display of (normal) Ia on B cells is also affected by HCQ. Change in Ia display could reduce effective interaction between antigen-presenting cells and amplifying intermediaries, i.e., T- and B-lymphocytes. Interference with these processes may therefore also be involved in HCQ immunosuppressant activity.

The immune cells that are most sensitive to HCQ are memory B cells, i.e., cells that have previously undergone encoding for a specific antigen. Memory B cells do not produce antibodies themselves, rather they bind antigen for which they are encoded and process and present it similarly to macrophages, i.e., they function as antigen-presenting cells during rechallenge. Memory B cell function can be depressed by levels of HCQ as low as 10 pM (10×10^{-12} M), or 10,000 times lower than required for most of the effects previously discussed. An exact role for memory B cells, and thus inhibition of them by HCQ, in RA is currently speculative but highly intriguing.

Mechanisms of Side Effects

Before beginning any description of side effects of the antimalarials, it is worthy of note that children are exquisitely sensitive, and death due to antimalarial treatment is a real possibility. The mechanism of the enhanced sensitivity is not known.

The range of side effects of HCQ is broad, and although exact mechanisms are mostly unknown, the concentration ranges for many have been documented. As stated previously, most anti-rheumatic doses produce plasma levels of approximately 1 μM (0.8–2.0 μM). Reversible side effects, including diplopia, dizziness, nausea, headache, skin rashes, and itching, have a threshold as low as 0.5–1.0 μM; however, in one study, no such side effects appeared at concentrations less than or equal to 1.25 μM, and 80% occurred at concentrations greater than 2.5 μM. Cardiovascular effects probably occur only in overdose (plasma levels greater than 3 μM) and may include hypotension, increased heart rate, and some prolongation of the QRS interval.

As indicated previously, HCQ has a very high affinity for melanin. In addition, melanin has a high capacity for HCQ. The retina (choroid, ciliary body), with its high melanin content, therefore accumulates very significant quantities of drug during chronic administration. Accumulation in the retina is associated with occurrence of visual difficulties, including blindness. The occurrence of retinopathies correlates with daily dose as well as with plasma levels: At 1 μM, a recommended 24-hour plasma maximum, no retinal damage occurred in a population with a 60% response rate, although recommended doses of chloroquine of 250 mg/day can give higher values (≤ 1.25 μM). Vision also may be impaired by drug deposition in the cornea, although the relative frequency of such deposits is unclear.

EXPECTATIONS AND DOSAGE SCHEDULES IN RA

The antimalarials are among the least effective and the least toxic of the slow-acting agents, and their efficacy is largely a matter of opinion. Early uncontrolled observations in RA suggested very good results; responses in the controlled studies were somewhat less impressive, but they were still comparable to other slow-acting drugs; and in the subsequent experience of many clinicians, response rates have been quite unimpressive. It is probably fair to suggest that these drugs are about as effective as auranofin; however, in certain SLE skin lesions, much better responses can be expected.

Initial doses of 400 mg/day of HCQ are usually recommended for RA. No response should be expected before two to three months, and the drug should not be considered a failure before six months of therapy. For patients who appear to be responding at six months, the daily dose can be reduced to 200 mg/day and continued indefinitely. If the disease appears to worsen during the maintenance period, the dose can again be increased to 400 mg/day for a few months or until improvement again becomes apparent. Larger initial doses (600 mg/day) are recommended by the manufacturer, but there is little evidence to support the benefits of the larger doses, which probably significantly increase the risk of toxicity.

Because the most serious side effect of antimalarial therapy is a maculopathy, toxicity monitoring consists of an ophthalmologic examination before the drug is given and every six months during therapy or at the discretion of the ophthalmologist. No routine laboratory studies are necessary.

CLINICAL ASPECTS OF SIDE EFFECTS

Although a number of potential side effects of antimalarial therapy exist, few are actually encountered in practice, though they might be more common if larger doses were used. Most of these reactions are thought to be more frequent with chloroquine than with HCQ. They are listed in Table 4-7. The length of this list reflects, in part, the several decades that these drugs have been available and their use in patients with malaria.

The relatively common minor reactions frequently respond to a temporary interruption of therapy or to temporary reductions in dose. The uncommon minor reactions, such as pigmentary changes, most often occur with prolonged therapy and are often asymptomatic. The major reactions most often reflect larger doses than those recommended here. Leukopenia and aplastic anemia are so unlikely with HCQ that routine laboratory monitoring has not been widely employed, but periodic complete blood counts might be prudent. Serious cardiac or neuromuscular symptoms should result in drug withdrawal, at least until the cause of the problem is established.

The most dreaded complication of antimalarial therapy is retinopathy, reflecting deposition of the drug in the macula. It can result in loss of vision, which has been reported to progress even after the drug was withdrawn. The incidence of the lesion is unclear but seems to be considerably less than 1%/year. The lesion is best detected by funduscopic examination and visual field testing, particularly with a small red test object. Patients should be evaluated by a knowledgeable ophthalmologist before antimalarial therapy is begun, and about every six months thereafter. The ophthalmologist might determine that more frequent evaluations are necessary.

Table 4-7. Reported side effects of chloroquine and hydroxychloroquine

Relatively common minor symptoms
  Abdominal discomfort
  Nausea and vomiting
  Diarrhea
  Anorexia
  Headache
  Lassitude
  Irritability
  Minor visual disturbances
  Vestibular disturbances
  Tinnitus
Uncommon minor reactions
  Skin and hair dyspigmentation
  Nail pigmentation
  Dermatitis
  Exacerbation of psoriasis
Uncommon major reactions
  Leukopenia
  Aplastic anemia
  Toxic psychosis
  Seizures
  Neuromyopathy
  Polyneuropathy
  Cardiomyopathy
  Retinopathy

CLINICAL INDICATIONS AND CONTRAINDICATIONS

In addition to malaria, the antimalarials (HCQ at least) are indicated for adult RA, discoid LE and SLE. HCQ is often chosen as the first slow-acting agent in RA. Children appear to be more sensitive to the toxic effects of the antimalarials, but there is some experience with these drugs in juvenile RA; uncontrolled observations suggest benefits, but one controlled study did not.

HCQ is FDA approved for use in SLE, and there is now evidence for beneficial effects on some of the minor extracutaneous manifestations, such as arthralgias and non-specific systemic symptoms. Controlled studies addressing this issue have also suggested that maintenance HCQ might prevent disease flares. It is very apparent that discoid skin lesions, whether primary or as a part of SLE, may respond rapidly and often dramatically to antimalarials. This has been appreciated for almost 100 years. Other skin lesions of SLE, especially subacute cutaneous lupus, may also respond. The overall response rate for lupus skin lesions is in the range of 60–80%. Dosage schedules are similar to those used for RA, but the onset of action is more rapid and maintenance doses can usually be established in less than six months.

Anecdotal reports suggest that antimalarials may benefit psoriatic arthritis, but they may also exacerbate the psoriasis. Too few experiences exist to suggest any other rheumatic disease indications.

Antimalarials are contraindicated in patients with prior serious reactions to any 4-aminoquinoline compound and pre-existing macular disease. They should not be prescribed for a rheumatic disorder in pregnant women. Reduced doses should be used in patients with renal insufficiency.

EXPENSE

A month of 400 mg/day of Plaquenil will cost the patient about $54. Assuming an ophthalmologic examination costs $100, the first six months of therapy will total $524, counting both the initial and the six-month eye examination. On 200 mg/day maintenance, the yearly cost will be about the same as that for the first six months—$524; therefore, antimalarials are among the least expensive of the slow-acting therapies in RA.

Methotrexate

The use of methotrexate (MTX) in RA currently enjoys such enthusiasm that one editorialist has referred to the early 1990s as the "methotrexate era." A folate antagonist and forerunner of MTX, aminopterin, was first used successfully in RA in the early 1950s, and MTX was reported to be effective in RA and psoriatic arthritis 10 years later. Few observations were reported over the next decade, but it became apparent to the dermatologists treating psoriasis with the drug that low doses given on a weekly basis minimized toxicity. The weekly dosage schedule was derived on the basis of skin turnover time, which is irrelevant to RA, but that schedule was adopted by rheumatologists as they began more widespread studies in RA in the 1970s. Several controlled clinical trials in the 1980s clearly documented the efficacy and relative safety of MTX in RA, and it was FDA approved for use in that disease in 1989.

MTX is available as 2.5-mg tablets and in a parenteral solution containing 25 mg/ml. It is widely assumed that oral and parenteral forms of the drug are interchangeable, though that has not been clearly established. Since FDA approval, oral MTX has been marketed as Rheumatrex and is provided in Dose Packs providing a month's supply of the drug for patients taking 5, 7.5, 10, 12.5, or 15 mg/week. Each weekly dose has its own dose pack.

BASIC PHARMACOLOGY

General Properties and Biochemical Mechanism

MTX is an analog of folic acid, and its basic action is that of an antimetabolite. For reference, the structures of MTX and folic acid are shown in Fig. 4-7. MTX is a weak organic acid that is primarily in an ionized, very water soluble form above pH 7. MTX is relatively insoluble below pH 7. In doses used orally in the therapy of RA, almost complete absorption occurs. Subsequent to absorption, the drug is widely distributed and actively taken up into cells via the transporter for 5-methyltetrahydrofolate (5-methyl-FH$_4$), for which 5-formyl-FH$_4$ (leucovorin) is also a ligand. Significant levels of MTX are found in synovial fluid and surrounding cells.

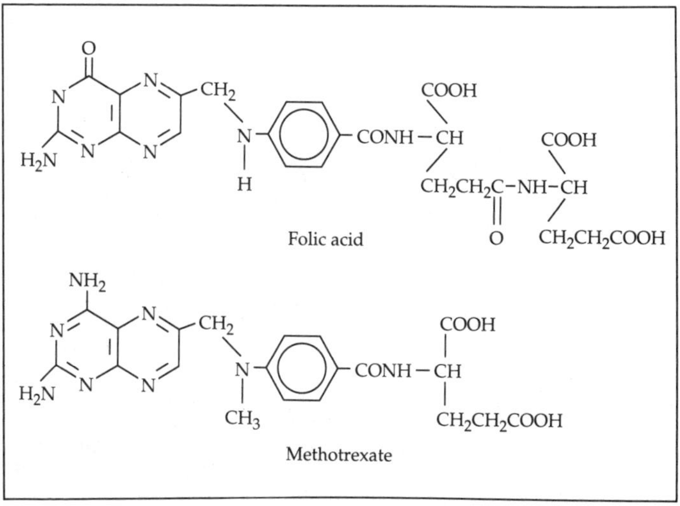

Fig. 4-7. Structures of folic acid and its antimetabolite analog, methotrexate.

Once inside cells, MTX can be polyglutamylated, with one to four glutamyl residues possible and two common. The polyglutamylated forms are too large for diffusion and are also charged; they are thus trapped inside cells and accumulation can occur. Different types of cells demonstrate differing rates and extents of polyglutamylation of MTX: Those with low capacity accumulate less MTX and are less likely to develop toxic effects; cells with high capacity and rate will accumulate significant quantities of MTX and are more likely to develop toxicity. Fortunately, from the standpoint of side effects, both bone marrow and gastrointestinal epithelial cells are slow-polyglutamylating tissues. In contrast, lymphoblasts are rapid poly-glutamylators.

The actual site of action of MTX is the enzyme dihydrofolate (FH_2) reductase, which converts FH_2 to FH_4, the active methylene carrier (one carbon donor) for synthesis of pyrimidines, e.g., thymidine. Ultimately, thymidine deficiency leads to decreased DNA synthesis and, if continued long enough, cell death. Since MTX also affects RNA and protein synthesis, it can be classified with azathioprine/6MP, i.e., MTX is an S-phase (proliferation)–specific, self-limited antimetabolite (see Fig. 4-5, previous section, for growth cycle diagram).

MTX is not metabolized to any extent, although small amounts of 7-OH-MTX may be formed. 7-OH-MTX is less toxic, but even more insoluble than MTX and thus has the potential to add to renal side effects of MTX. MTX is renally eliminated by both filtration and active secretion via the tubular organic acid (organic anion) transporter. Elimination kinetics are characteristic of multiple (three) compartments; the early phase half-life is about an hour, whereas the longest phase half-life may be up to 10 hours. The length of the latter may reflect slow release from cells as well as a small contribution from enterohepatic circulation.

Mechanisms of Immunosuppression

As stated before, lymphocyte precursors are more sensitive than myeloid precursors (in bone marrow) or gastrointestinal stem cells. Implied in this is the possibility of decreased T- or B-lymphocyte proliferation; however, in patients treated with MTX for RA, no decreases in circulating numbers of T or B cells, or in their relative ratios, are observed.

B cell function is influenced, however, and results in decreased immunoglobulin levels and decreased levels of RF. Much of this appears due to effects on monocytes/macrophages: Macrophage activation is inhibited, monocyte influx into synovial tissue is inhibited, PGE_2 release is inhibited, and, perhaps most importantly, IL-1 release is inhibited (details of IL-1 release, effects, and role in inflammation can be found in Chapter 3; additional reference to IL-1 occurs throughout this chapter as well). Since IL-1 is the signal to T-lymphocytes (helper) to release IL-2, or lymphocyte growth factor, inhibition of IL-1 alone could account for much of MTX's immunosuppressive action.

The possibility has been raised that MTX might act to reduce a specific T cell population that is involved in the ongoing autoimmune response. The suggestion is based on data for an experimentally induced, MTX-responsive arthritis caused by a low molecular weight, basic protein mitogen elaborated by *Mycobacterium arthritides*. In *M. arthritides* arthritis, a sub-population of T-lymphocytes that recognizes **both** the mycobacterium **and** proteoglycans in joint cartilage can be isolated. These dual recognition cells may compose less than 2% of the total T population, suggesting that MTX-induced reduction in this population could not be detected easily. Whether such a scenario applies in RA is unknown but is certainly of ongoing interest.

Mechanisms of Side Effects

With any agent that inhibits cell replication, side effects related to bone marrow suppression (leukopenia, thrombocytopenia), damage to gastrointestinal mucosa (nausea, anorexia, diarrhea, and vomiting; mucositis, stomatitis) and skin (rashes, alopecia) can occur; however, at the low doses at which MTX is used in RA, these effects are uncommon, in the order of 5%. As pointed out previously, MTX is relatively insoluble below pH 7, and it is renally excreted; these two features explain the occasional occurrence of intrarenal precipitation of drug and the fact that increased urinary volume and pH are helpful. Again, however, this effect is not usual for low doses of MTX.

Two serious side effects can occur even with low-dose therapy, namely pneumonitis and cirrhosis and hepatic fibrosis. MTX pneumonitis is often accompanied by eosinophilia and may be a hypersensitivity response. This is very reminiscent of the "gold lung" previously described. Importantly, the pneumonitis can proceed to fibrosis if unrecognized or if therapy is not withdrawn, or both. Liver damage similarly can proceed to cirrhosis and fibrosis if unrecognized or if therapy is not withdrawn, or both. One suggestion is that intermittent therapy is less likely to cause liver damage than continuous therapy. An additional effect that may accompany chronic low-dose therapy is **osteoporosis**. The mechanism(s) is unknown but perhaps may reflect some sensitivity of osteoblasts to MTX.

In closing details of toxicity, it should be noted that folate deficiency can predispose to toxicity occurrence, for obvious reasons if considered. Also, decreased or delayed clearance of the drug can lead to unexpected toxicity.

Several drug interactions have been suggested for MTX, but these seem to be mainly of theoretical interest. These include protein-binding displacement of MTX by salicylate, sulfonamides, and other highly protein-bound drugs and decreased renal secretion of MTX in the presence of probenecid. Since MTX may also undergo renal reabsorption, it would be of interest to know whether this occurs via the same uptake mechanism as uric acid and whether probenecid could analogously decrease reabsorption.

EXPECTATIONS AND DOSAGE SCHEDULES IN RA

It has been debated whether MTX should be classified as a SAARD since its onset of action is typically more rapid than the other drugs in this group. Beneficial effects are often apparent within a month of beginning an effective dose. This rapid onset of action is one of the reasons for the current enthusiasm among rheumatologists for MTX. In several placebo-controlled and comparative studies, the efficacy of the drug appears to be similar to parenteral gold and the other more effective SAARDs. In several observations, however, the drop-out rate for lack of efficacy has been impressively low—perhaps around 10%, suggesting a response rate in the range of 90%, clearly superior to the other slow-acting agents. A response rate of 90% may be somewhat inflated, but many clinicians do feel that MTX is more likely than the other slow-acting drugs to result in an acceptable clinical response, again adding to the general enthusiasm for its use. No evidence exists, however, to show that MTX is more likely than other drugs in its class to induce a complete remission.

Assuming no relative contraindications (such as renal insufficiency), MTX is usually begun in a dose of 7.5 mg/week. It is a matter of opinion as to how often dose adjustments should be made, but any suggestion of improvement with the initial or a lower dose after a month should delay the decision at least another month to allow for maximum improvement. No apparent response to 7.5 mg/week after one or two months should lead to a 2.5-mg increment for another month or two. The dose can be adjusted upward in this fashion until an acceptable clinical response is established or a total weekly dose of 15 mg is reached. If no benefits are apparent two months after beginning the 15 mg/week program, the drug probably should be considered a failure, though some rheumatologists would proceed to 17.5 mg or even 20 mg/week before abandoning it. Higher doses are clearly associated with more toxicity, but a 17.5- or 20-mg/week trial might be justified in patients who had failed to respond to all other slow-acting agents. Whatever weekly dosages are used, the tablets can be taken all at once or divided in two or three doses 12 hours apart. The latter approach may reduce gastrointestinal side effects and is usually recommended with the larger doses.

Once the weekly dose required to produce a satisfactory response is established, it is not necessarily continued indefinitely. A number of patients will continue to improve with time, and downward dose adjustments should be attempted to seek the lowest one effective. More likely there will be gradual worsening with time, and most of these patients appear to respond to gradual increments in dose. Consequently there is no one maintenance dose of MTX in RA; it varies and is adjusted according to the clinical response. Long-term observations of MTX therapy in RA have suggested an impressively high patient retention rate when this type of program is followed, further adding to the general enthusiasm for the drug.

Although not specifically recommended by the manufacturer or specifically approved by the FDA, the parenteral form of the drug is widely used in the same doses as the oral preparation. Exact equivalence has not been clearly documented but is widely assumed. Advantages of the parenteral preparation are fewer apparent side effects (again not clearly documented) and considerably less expense. It has been shown that absorption from subcutaneous administration is similar to that from the intramuscular route. Consequently it might be permissible to allow patients to give themselves subcutaneous injections at home.

Meanwhile toxicity monitoring consists of periodic complete blood counts, usually every 2–4 weeks, and tests for hepatotoxicity, usually every two or three months. Recent evidence suggests that the addition of folic acid in a dose of 1 mg/day significantly reduces MTX toxicity without interfering with its beneficial effects. This program probably should be recommended to the patient.

CLINICAL ASPECTS OF SIDE EFFECTS

Just how serious are MTX side effects is the subject of current debate, with some authorities arguing that it is among the safest of the slow-acting agents. It is becoming apparent that the experience with the drug in patients with psoriasis cannot be entirely transposed to the RA population taking it. Clearly the lowest effective dose given once a week minimizes toxicity; it appears that folate supplementation further reduces the risk of side effects; and the bparenteral route of administration may help protect against some of the reactions. But serious concerns still exist and are justified, especially considering that the widespread use of MTX in patients with RA is a relatively recent phenomenon.

The significant reactions are listed in Table 4-8. Only those pertinent to the use of the drug in rheumatic diseases will be addressed. The toxicity profile resulting from high doses used to treat malignancy is quite different and not relevant to this discussion.

The very common gastrointestinal symptoms often can be abolished or made tolerable by dividing the weekly doses or by changing to a parenteral route of administration. Dermatologic manifestations

Table 4-8. Side effects reported from low-dose weekly methotrexate

Common and usually not serious
  Nausea and vomiting
  Abdominal discomfort
  Diarrhea
  Abnormal liver tests
  Macrocytosis
  Stomatitis
  Pruritus/dermatitis
  Alopecia
  Headache and memory impairment
Common and potentially serious
  Thrombocytopenia
  Leukopenia
  Pancytopenia
Uncommon and potentially lethal
  Pulmonary infiltrates with hypoxemia
  Hepatic cirrhosis
  Acute hepatic failure

and stomatitis may respond to withholding the drug for one or two weeks and then restarting it in lower doses, gradually returning to the original schedule. These side effects may also respond to topical therapy. Modest disturbances in the liver tests may not require any action since they do not necessarily predict significant hepatic damage. They are often disconcerting, however, and may cease to be a problem if the dose is reduced or if the parenteral route of administration is used. Macrocytosis is not itself a problem, but it may predict more serious hematologic toxicity; it can be minimized by folate supplementation.

The hemocytopenias, especially leukopenia, may occur at any time during the course of therapy. They may be partially preventable by folate supplementation and usually respond to temporary interruption of therapy followed by a reduction in dose. These reactions have often been associated with accidental overdosage or standard doses given to patients with renal insufficiency.

The pulmonary reaction is one of the most dreaded complications of MTX therapy. It was reported in 3% of RA patients taking the drug in one experience, but it is probably not that common. Underlying rheumatoid lung disease may predispose to the reaction, and it may occur at any time during the course of therapy. It typically presents relatively acutely with cough, fever, and dyspnea. Diffuse infiltrates are seen on chest x-ray and hypoxemia is present. Deaths have been reported, but the reaction apparently responds to high-dose corticosteroid therapy. Residual lung damage has been found in survivors of the reaction. A base-line chest x-ray is recommended before beginning MTX, both for future reference and to determine if pre-existing lung disease is present. If evidence of rheumatoid lung disease exists, the therapy should be reconsidered. Patients should be warned of the reaction and told to promptly report any symptoms suggesting it. MTX should not be taken in the presence of pulmonary symptoms until they are evaluated by a physician.

Hepatic reactions, especially cirrhosis, have been a major focus of the concerns over MTX toxicity since it was first used in RA, but reassuring data are beginning to surface. These concerns derive primarily from the psoriasis experience in which cumulative doses as low as 2 gm or less were associated with irreversible hepatic fibrosis. Although this remains a major concern in patients with psoriasis treated with MTX, series of liver biopsies from RA patients with cumulative doses as large as 6–8 gm have usually failed to show either significant fibrosis or alarming degrees of hepatic necrosis or inflammation; however, the possibility of cirrhosis cannot be entirely discounted yet. Routine liver biopsies in RA patients after cumulative doses of 4–6 gm of MTX are still recommended by some authorities, and this recommendation should be discussed with the patient. Abnormalities in the liver tests during the course of therapy do not predict hepatic fibrosis, and some psoriatic patients have had cirrhosis found on biopsy with no preceding laboratory abnormalities. This raises the question of what to do with abnormal liver tests found routinely in the course of laboratory monitoring. The answer is not known, but many cautious clinicians prefer to try to normalize them with adjustments in dose or dosage form. General agreement exists that MTX should not be given to patients who abuse alcohol or who have known pre-existing liver disease. In patients with psoriasis, obesity and diabetes mellitus appeared to be risk factors for hepatotoxicity.

Recently a few cases of acute hepatic failure have been reported in RA patients taking methotrexate. A definite causal relationship has not been clearly established, but clinical hepatitis or markedly abnormal liver tests should result in immediate and permanent withdrawal of MTX therapy.

It is relatively clear that MTX is not oncogenic and does not permanently impair sexual function, but it is teratogenic and should not be taken during pregnancy.

Concerns have been raised that NSAIDs, including the salicylates, could enhance MTX toxicity by displacing the drug from its protein-binding sites. No clinical data support these concerns, and NSAIDs have been used routinely in patients taking MTX; however, enhanced toxicity has been reported with the concomitant use of other drugs with antifolate activity (trimethoprim and sulfamethoxazole).

Measures aimed at minimizing or preventing MTX toxicity are summarized in Table 4-9. If these guidelines are followed, it is likely that this drug will prove to be one of the safest of the slow-acting agents.

CLINICAL INDICATIONS AND CONTRAINDICATIONS

In addition to malignancy, MTX is FDA approved only for severe psoriasis and severe adult RA. As yet too few data exist to support its safety and efficacy in juvenile RA, but at least one controlled trial in the polyarticular form of the disease is in progress.

Among the rheumatic diseases other than RA, MTX is probably most often used for psoriatic arthritis, though its efficacy in this condition has not been documented clearly in controlled clinical trials. It should be reserved for patients with either severe skin disease or

Table 4-9. Measures to prevent or minimize weekly low-dose methotrexate toxicity

Absolute contraindications
  Alcohol abuse
  Known liver disease
  Pregnancy
  Anticipated pregnancy (immediate)
  Severe lung disease
  Severe renal insufficiency
  Pancytopenia
  Malignancy
  Human immunodeficiency virus infection

Relative contraindications
  Alcohol use
  Obesity
  Diabetes mellitus
  Mild renal insufficiency (indicates reduced dose)
  Pre-existing cytopenias
  Chronic infection
  History of malignancy
  Peptic ulcer disease
  Anticoagulant therapy

Pretreatment studies
  Complete blood count
  Liver tests
  Chest x-ray
  Renal function
  Pulmonary function (?)
  Human immunodeficiency virus test (if risk factors present)

Advise patients to avoid
  More than one (or two?) alcoholic drinks/day
  Pregnancy
  Other antifolate or cytotoxic drugs

Advise patients to report
  Cough, fever, dyspnea
  Jaundice
  Nausea, vomiting, diarrhea
  Abnormal bleeding
  Severe infections
  Mouth sores

Perform
  Complete blood counts every 3–4 wks
  Tests of liver function every 6–8 wks
  Liver biopsy after total cumulative dose of 4–6 gm (controversial)

Prescribe
  Folic acid, 1 mg/day

progressive erosive polyarthritis unresponsive to NSAIDs. An indefinite commitment to the therapy need not be made. Dosage schedules are similar to those used in RA and similar toxicity can be expected, except that cirrhosis is probably more likely. A pretreatment liver biopsy has been recommended, and an additional biopsy should be considered after a cumulative dose of 2 gm.

Though there are no controlled studies, MTX has been used for over 20 years in patients with polymyositis, usually those unresponsive to or requiring continuing large doses of corticosteroids. The drug has most often been given parenterally in a weekly schedule, but in doses larger than those recommended for RA, typically 20–50 mg/week. Its efficacy has seldom been questioned, but the large doses involved increase the likelihood of toxicity. Smaller weekly doses might be used to reduce corticosteroid requirements, but, again, no published data exist to support the usefulness of this practice.

Numerous anecdotal reports suggest that MTX might benefit the more severe forms of Reiter's syndrome, and preliminary reports suggest that it might be useful in controlling the symptoms of active SLE. Other uses in rheumatology are certain to be explored as more is learned about its antirheumatic effects. Meanwhile the drug is being investigated in nonrheumatic inflammatory diseases such as asthma. It appears to have a promising future.

Contraindications are listed in Table 4-9. Mild renal insufficiency should result in a reduction in weekly dosage, beginning with 2.5 or 5.0 mg. The association of Reiter's syndrome with the acquired immunodeficiency syndrome lead to the recognition that MTX can severely exacerbate the latter. Human immunodeficiency virus (HIV) testing is recommended before MTX administration if any risk factors for HIV infection are present.

EXPENSE

Pretreatment evaluation will cost the patient about $100 (chest x-ray, complete blood count, and chemistry profile). Monthly Rheumatrex Dose Packs cost about $35 for 7.5 mg/week; $45 for 10 mg/week; $55 for 12.5 mg/week; and $65 for 15 mg/week. considering a complete blood count to be $15 and to be done monthly and a liver profile to be $23, and assuming an effective dose of 15 mg/week, arrived at after increasing the dose by 2.5 mg every two months, the first six months of therapy will cost the patient a total of $529. If the 15 mg/week is continued indefinitely, the annual cost will be $1098. If the weekly dose were 10 mg (as it more often is), the annual cost would be $768.

A 2-ml vial containing 25 mg/ml or 50 mg of MTX costs the patient about $20. Assuming no charges for the injections, a six-month dose-finding program as outlined before using the parenteral preparation would cost the patient $100 for the pretreatment tests, $159 for laboratory monitoring, and only $96 for the drug for a total of $355. Annual cost of 15 mg/week maintenance would be reduced to $630 ($318 for the lab and $312 for the drug). Obviously the cost-effectiveness of the parenteral route would be lost if the patient were charged for the injections. For any dosage schedule or route of administration employed, about $4/month can be added to the total charges if folate supplementation is elected.

Sulfasalazine

Sulfasalazine is the conjugate of 5-aminosalicylic acid (5-ASA) and sulfapyridine. Its history is colorful. In the late 1930s and early

1940s, when the drug was created and first used, the combination of an antibiotic (only sulfonamides were available) and an anti-inflammatory agent seemed ideal for the treatment of RA, then widely regarded as an infectious disease. Consequently sulfasalazine was specifically designed with RA in mind. Initial trials in that disease seemed successful, but a rather negative result when the drug was compared to parenteral gold lead to almost complete loss of interest in its antirheumatic effects. Later, of course, it was found to be effective in ulcerative colitis, keeping it available worldwide. In the late 1970s and early 1980s, small successful trials in RA were published, leading to a number of placebo-controlled and comparative studies that have clearly documented the efficacy of the drug as a slow-acting agent in RA. It is widely used for that purpose in Europe but has not yet (1991) been FDA approved for use in RA in this country. A particularly interesting aspect of the antirheumatic effects of the drug concerns the evidence that it is the sulfapyridine, and not the 5-ASA, that is effective, leading to further speculations on the etiology of RA; however, the mechanism of action remains unknown.

Sulfasalazine is available in 500-mg tablets as Azulfidine or it is available generically. Azulfidine EN-Tabs are an enteric-coated form of the drug, and enteric-coated generic preparations are also available, as is an oral suspension.

BASIC PHARMACOLOGY

General Properties and Mechanisms

As mentioned in the introduction, sulfasalazine has been in successful use for other disorders, particularly ulcerative colitis, for a considerable time. Its use in RA is less lengthy and therefore data supporting mechanisms are sparse. The following brief discussion will include some observations from proposed gastrointestinal mechanisms that may apply to therapy of RA.

Sulfasalazine is a diazo conjugate of 5-ASA, which has some anti-inflammatory activity, and sulfapyridine, a sulfonamide antibiotic (Fig. 4-8). The intact drug is poorly absorbed after oral administration ($\leq 30\%$). Orally absorbed drug is reduced in the liver and its components liberated. Intact drug in the gut lumen also can be broken down to its components in the upper gastrointestinal tract, after which sulfapyridine is rapidly absorbed. Sulfapyridine is a short-acting, water-soluble sulfonamide antibiotic; its mode of action in microbes is inhibition of para-aminobenzoic acid incorporation into folic acid.

Although 5-ASA is absorbed, high concentrations are found in feces. Because of the latter, and because of the anti-inflammatory and other effects of 5-ASA, efficacy of sulfasalazine in ulcerative colitis often has been ascribed to its content of 5-ASA. Indeed, considerable controversy has concerned which entity, i.e., intact parent or one or the other component, or a combination, is responsible for sulfasalazine's efficacy in ulcerative colitis. The same controversy continues for its use in RA.

Both sulfasalazine and 5-ASA, a salicylate, can, at sufficient concentrations, limit formation of eicosanoids (see Chapter 2 for details

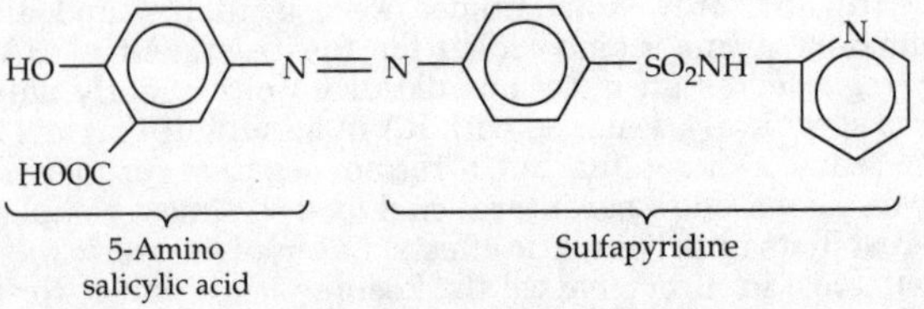

Fig. 4-8. Structure of salicylazosulfapyridine.

of arachidonic acid metabolism), including LTB_4 and prostaglandins. These data are from in vitro studies of colonic mucosal cells and may or may not extend to neutrophils or monocytes. The drug concentrations required to inhibit mucosal release of eicosanoids are in the millimolar (≈ 3.5 mM; 3.5×10^{-3} M) range, i.e., very high. Other in vitro data support an interaction between 5-ASA and oxygen radicals (e.g., superoxide), i.e., 5-ASA may act as a radical scavenger. The radical scavenging action is suggested to account for normalization of lipid peroxide levels in bowel biopsy specimens of ulcerative colitis patients treated with sulfasalazine.

In other in vitro studies, sulfasalazine itself was demonstrated to inhibit proliferative responses of mixed peripheral lymphocyte populations or of purified B-lymphocytes. Again, however, relatively high concentrations of drug were required (c 0.3 mM). Decreased B cell production of immunoglobulins, and also IgM-RF, were observed using cells from RA patients, and this effect was obtained at concentrations $10\times$ lower than required for antiproliferative effects (c 30–65 μM), or in the range expected subsequent to usual doses (peak $\approx$ 30–40 μM after a single 2-gm dose). The components of sulfasalazine, 5-ASA and sulfapyridine, had no antiproliferative effects nor did they decrease immunoglobulin production at equivalent concentrations. In vivo administration of sulfasalazine has been shown to reduce the numbers of circulating activated lymphocytes. Cells taken from the same treated patients showed decreased mitogenic responses to lectin (Concanavalin A) stimulation. In vitro cell exposure to either 5-ASA or sulfapyridine likewise inhibited lectin-induced responses.

Support for an immunomodulatory effect of sulfasalazine also comes from the observation that it can enhance effects of cyclosporine (on graft rejection). Clearly, additional data supporting both efficacy in RA and mechanisms are highly desirable.

Mechanisms of Side Effects and Drug Interactions

The side effects of sulfasalazine are common to most sulfonamides and include gastrointestinal effects (nausea, vomiting, stomatitis, pain), CNS effects (headache, dizziness), hypersensitivity reactions (skin rashes, photosensitization, pneumonitis with eosinophilia, fever, arthralgias), and blood dyscrasias (thrombocytopenia, leukopenia, aplastic anemia).

Mechanisms are generally not known for most of the aforementioned side effects. One study in an animal model suggests that complement activation may occur simultaneously with immunosuppression by sulfasalazine; complement activation was proposed as a mechanism for drug-induced hypersensitivity reactions, but this suggestion requires additional documentation, particularly in humans.

Because sulfapyridine acts to prevent microbial synthesis of folic acid, and because humans are entirely dependent on folic acid produced by their gastrointestinal flora, macrocytic anemia can occur during sulfasalazine therapy. Supplementation with folic acid is preventive. Glucose 6-phosphate dehydrogenase–deficient red cells may undergo hemolysis subsequent to sulfasalazine/component exposure.

The only drug interaction of significance for sulfasalazine appears to be a sulfasalazine-induced decrease in digoxin absorption. Increases in digoxin dose may be required. Theoretically, interactions by protein-binding displacement for other highly protein-bound drugs are possible.

EXPECTATIONS AND DOSAGE SCHEDULES IN RA

Published open and controlled trials have involved variable dosage schedules, making it difficult to generalize concerning the effectiveness of sulfasalazine in RA, but in doses of 2–3 gm/day, it is probably less effective than parenteral gold and perhaps about as effective as auranofin. Some comparative trials, however, have suggested a response rate similar to that of parenteral gold and D-penicillamine.

When used for RA, sulfasalazine is probably most often given in a dose of 2 gm/day in four divided doses, making it somewhat inconvenient. It has been recommended that lower doses be given initially, gradually increasing to 2 gm/day in order to minimize side effects. At the 2-gm dose, responses begin to become apparent at about two months, but at least four and preferably six months of therapy are required before the drug can be considered a failure. If no benefits are apparent after four to six months of 2 gm/day, the dose might be increased to 3 gm/day for an additional two months before the drug is abandoned. Successful therapy is continued indefinitely. Too few experiences exist to suggest an approach to late drug failures.

Meanwhile toxicity monitoring consists of periodic complete blood counts, perhaps biweekly initially and then every eight weeks if no reactions occur early in the course of therapy. Periodic liver tests have also been advocated, though hepatitis from the drug is rare. The manufacturers also recommend periodic urinalyses, though renal reactions have been extremely rare in patients taking the drug for RA.

CLINICAL ASPECTS OF SIDE EFFECTS

Of course, the long-term experience with sulfasalazine has been in patients with ulcerative colitis often taking doses larger than those generally used for RA, and the toxicity profile in these patients might be different from the experience in RA. A large experience with the drug in the latter disease has been published suggesting that as many as 26% of RA patients taking sulfasalazine will stop the drug because of side effects, but most of the reactions reported were mild or trivial. It is relatively clear that the majority of side effects tend to occur in the first few months of therapy, suggesting more intensive toxicity monitoring early in the course of treatment.

By far the most common side effects are upper gastrointestinal symptoms: abdominal discomfort, nausea, and vomiting. These are more likely in patients with the slow-acetylator phenotype. These symptoms can be minimized by using the enteric-coated tablets, which probably should be prescribed routinely. The second most common group of reactions are mucocutaneous, largely nonspecific maculopapular or urticarial rashes. Depending on their severity, these side effects may or may not necessitate permanent withdrawal of therapy.

Potentially more serious are the hematologic effects that occur in less than 1% of sulfasalazine-treated patients. Leukopenia is the most common, but thrombocytopenia and anemias due to bone marrow aplasia have been reported. Sulfasalazine may impair folate absorption leading to a megaloblastic anemia, and the drug may precipitate hemolysis in subjects with glucose 6-phosphate dehydrogenase deficiency. Any significant hemocytopenia encountered during routine toxicity monitoring should result in interruption of therapy at least until another cause can be established; if no other cause is established, the drug should be permanently discontinued.

Hepatitis, eosinophilic pneumonia, fibrosing alveolitis, and male infertility have also been reported with sulfasalazine therapy, primarily in patients with ulcerative colitis. Despite the toxicity withdrawal rate reported in some trials and despite the variety of side effects on record, sulfasalazine is widely regarded as one of the least toxic of the slow-acting agents.

CLINICAL INDICATIONS AND CONTRAINDICATIONS

Sulfasalazine is not yet FDA approved for any rheumatic disease but probably will be approved at least for use in adult RA. Several trials, some controlled, also suggest a role for the drug as a slow-acting agent in ankylosing spondylitis. Dosage schedules and response rates have been similar to those observed in RA. In three controlled clinical trials, symptoms, spinal mobility, and laboratory parameters improved more with sulfasalazine than with placebo. No interpretable published observations exist for sulfasalazine use in other rheumatic diseases.

Several reports have suggested that the addition of sulfasalazine to other slow-acting therapies (oral and parenteral gold and D-penicillamine) might result in further improvement in patients with RA, and a synergistic effect has even been suggested. Further studies will be required before this practice can be recommended, but it has been safe in the few reported trials.

Sulfasalazine is contraindicated in patients with a prior serious reaction to it and in patients with a sensitivity to sulfonamides or salicylates. It should be used with caution in subjects with a deficiency of glucose 6-phosphate dehydrogenase. It may be safe during pregnancy but is best avoided.

EXPENSE

Assuming a daily dose of 2 gm, a month's supply of Azulfidine En-Tabs will cost the patient about $32 and the generic enteric-coated preparations will be about $10 less. Considering laboratory monitoring to consist of a complete blood count monthly for the first six months and then every other month, the therapy could cost as little as $270 for the first six months, and then $402 annually, making it the least expensive of the slow-acting agents.

Cyclophosphamide

Although its efficacy in RA has been documented, cyclophosphamide is not usually considered a SAARD in that context. Because of its toxicity, it is usually used for more life-threatening conditions such as systemic vasculitis and severe SLE. Curiously the only nonmalignant disease for which the drug is FDA approved is corticosteroid-resistant "minimal change" nephrotic syndrome in children. Because of its toxicity, it will probably never be approved for active RA, but a number of other rheumatic conditions are sufficiently serious (or lethal) to justify its use, and an occasional patient with severe RA will respond only to it.

Cyclophosphamide is available in 25-mg and 50-mg tablets as Cytoxan and generically in various parenteral forms. It is used orally and intravenously for rheumatic conditions.

BASIC PHARMACOLOGY OF CYCLOPHOSPHAMIDE AND CHLORAMBUCIL

General Properties and Mechanisms

Although chlorambucil is discussed under a separate clinical applications section from cyclophosphamide, its basic pharmacology and mechanism of action are essentially identical to cyclophosphamide; therefore, some mention of it will be included here for simplicity and to emphasize the relationship between the two drugs.

Cyclophosphamide and chlorambucil belong to the group of drugs known as **nitrogen mustards**. The nitrogen mustards are used most frequently in therapy of neoplastic diseases. The parent molecules are inactive and must undergo (hepatic) microsomal oxidation before they are capable of the internal rearrangement required to become active alkylating agents. The structures of cyclophosphamide and chlorambucil, the reactive alkylating ethyleneimonium ion, and some conversions of cyclophosphamide to active metabolites are shown in Fig. 4-9.

It should be noted that each compound has two chloroethyl groups, each of which can form a reactive ion capable of attaching to nucleophilic targets (e.g., sulfhydryl, amino, phosphate, hydroxyl and carboxyl groups); therefore, these drugs can act as cross-linking

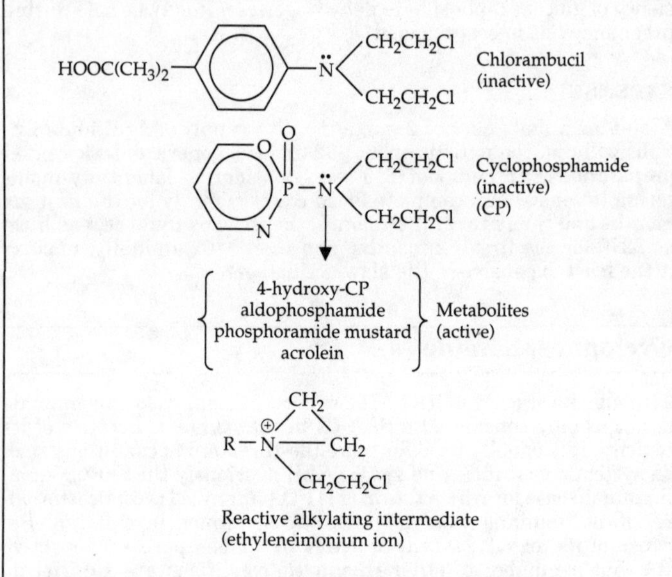

Fig. 4-9. Structures of two bifunctional alkylating agents, cyclophosphamide (CP) and chlorambucil. Both agents are inactive until converted to several metabolites (shown for CP); the metabolites can form the reactive alkylating intermediate (ethyleneimonium ion).

agents for macromolecules, including DNA, RNA, and proteins (e.g., enzymes). The order of sensitivity of the macromolecules is DNA > RNA > protein. DNA cross-linking can be between two strands via bonds between adjacent guanine bases or can also occur from DNA to adjacent proteins. The functional result of DNA cross-linking is lack of DNA replication and translation, and potentially cell death. For reference, cyclophosphamide is cycle specific, i.e., it acts on both cycling and intermitotic cells, although rapidly proliferating cells may be more affected. In contrast, previously mentioned cytotoxic drugs, azathioprine/6MP, and MTX, are phase (S-phase) specific.

Cyclophosphamide is well absorbed after oral administration. It is minimally plasma protein bound, although some of its active metabolites are bound to a greater degree ($\approx$ 50%). As mentioned, hepatic biotransformation must occur for the drug to be active; decreased hepatic function could reduce activation and effect. Cyclophosphamide and its metabolites, active and inactive, are eliminated via the kidney. There are two potential consequences of the route of elimination: Reduced renal function may prolong and intensify drug effect, and the urinary bladder is exposed to acrolein, one of the active metabolites that apparently produces the characteristic cystitis associated with cyclophosphamide use. Cystitis is reported to occur even with chronic low-dose therapy, although it is more common with higher doses.

Mechanisms of Immunosuppression

Cyclophosphamide therapy of RA produces significant reductions in B- and T-lymphocyte populations, to as low as 25% of pretreatment values. The relative proportions of B and T cells appear to be unchanged, however, although some reports of greater reductions in T cells have occurred.

In addition to effects on cell numbers, cyclophosphamide also affects function. Newly stimulated, rapidly proliferating B cells produce significantly less immunoglobulin subsequent to cyclophosphamide exposure. Curiously, IgE production may be augmented at the same time IgG is reduced. The latter has been attributed to selective removal of a subpopulation of T suppressor cells that ordinarily keep IgE production low. Notably, immunoglobulin levels decrease in cyclophosphamide-treated RA patients. Immunoglobulin reduction occurs by direct effect on B cells, rather than on T-helpers. In addition to reducing B cell immunoglobulin production, cyclophosphamide has been stated to decrease expression of immunoglobulin on cell surfaces.

Effects on T-lymphocytes are less clear, in terms of an overall picture. Generally, T-suppressors may be more sensitive than other T-populations, such that in some settings, cyclophosphamide can have immunoenhancing effects. The enhanced IgE production mentioned previously falls in this category. Immunoenhancement by removal of T-suppressors may be more likely when low doses are used, since inhibition of B cell function apparently occurs at higher drug levels. Immunoenhancement of the type observed with cyclophosphamide has not been reported for RA patients, however. A favorable result of the population-selective properties of cyclophosphamide is that global immunosuppression, with attendant complications, is less likely.

Mechanisms of Side Effects and Drug Interactions

The side effects of cyclophosphamide are fairly predictable and include bone marrow suppression (leukopenia more than thrombocytopenia), nausea, diarrhea, alopecia, cystitis, and possibly mutagenesis or carcinogenesis (or a combination of the latter two). The mechanism for cystitis production, i.e., acrolein irritation, is known. A specific agent to combat acrolein-induced cystitis (mesna; sodium 2-mercaptoethane sulfonate, a thiol) has been identified, mainly for coadministration with high doses of cyclophosphamide. Evidence exists that cyclophosphamide can also cause nephrotoxicity, even as severe as acute tubular necrosis, but the prevalence in low-dose regimens is not documented. An increased incidence of tumor development has not been indicated for low-dose cyclophosphamide.

Several drug interactions have been suggested, although their relevance to low-dose cyclophosphamide is questionable. Some are mentioned here for completeness. Cyclophosphamide **may** induce liver microsomal enzymes, and thus its own conversion to active products. Some increase in oral anticoagulant effect on withdrawal of cyclophosphamide may support an occasional interaction by this route. Cyclophosphamide activation, and inactivation, may be influenced by simultaneous administration of other inducers, e.g., phenobarbital. Allopurinol has been stated to interfere with drug excretion, and thus it may increase risk of bone marrow suppression by cyclophosphamide.

CLINICAL INDICATIONS AND CONTRAINDICATIONS

None of the conditions discussed in this section reflect FDA-approved indications for cyclophosphamide, but they do reflect either the results of controlled clinical trials or established patterns of usage among rheumatologists and nephrologists. The major rheumatic indications for cyclophosphamide are summarized in Table 4-10. For all of these conditions except active RA, high-dose corticosteroids are used initially with the cyclophosphamide, and then tapered as a satisfactory clinical response occurs. For most of these conditions, a clinical response begins to become apparent in two to four weeks, though active RA may require longer to respond. It is becoming apparent that pulse high-dose parenteral cyclophosphamide is better tolerated than the oral preparation taken on a regular basis, but this program has been systemically evaluated in only a few situations. It seems to be more effective than the oral route in lupus nephritis, but less effective in Wegener's granulomatosis.

It is somewhat ironic that the effectiveness of cyclophosphamide has been documented best in active RA, since most rheumatologists use it for that indication only as a last resort. The toxicity of the drug is a strong reason against its use in conditions that are not threatening life or vital organs. For patients with severe RA resistant to or intolerant of all other slow-acting therapies, the drug should be considered and offered to the patient. Unless the situation is extremely desperate, the lower doses (1 mg/kg/day) should be tried first. The safety of indefinite or long-term therapy is in serious doubt, and the question of withdrawing the drug from a patient who seems to need it will have to be addressed at some point months or years later. Depending on the dose used, toxicity monitoring will require at least a complete blood count and urinalysis every two to four weeks.

Currently rheumatologists and nephrologists are considerably enthusiastic for the use of high-dose pulses of intravenous cyclophosphamide in the more severe forms of lupus nephritis. Candidates for this therapy should at least have active and potentially reversible disease. A similar program is being widely used for active SLE affecting other organ systems as well, but no more than anecdotal reports support this practice, and it should be remembered that weeks may be required for a response to become apparent. Many of these disease flares abate on their own or respond to corticosteroids in less time. A number of different parenteral dosage schedules are being used in this country, mostly based on the protocol used by the National Institutes of Health for lupus nephritis. Usually about a gram is given every one to three months over the period of six months to a year.

Perhaps the most dramatically effective results of cyclophosphamide therapy occur in patients with systemic necrotizing vasculitis, especially Wegener's granulomatosis. Early therapy of these conditions with about 2–3 mg/kg/day of cyclophosphamide orally apparently results in permanent remissions in a significant number of these patients, making early diagnosis crucial. Duration of therapy required to produce a lasting remission is not clearly established, but the drug is usually given for at least a year. Preliminary observations suggest that high-dose pulses are not as effective as regular use of the oral preparation.

Contraindications to the use of cyclophosphamide are usually relative, but it would be prudent not to give the drug to rheumatic disease patients with a serious infection or a malignancy. A prior serious reaction to cyclophosphamide that did not respond to dose adjustments would also discourage further use of it.

CLINICAL ASPECTS OF SIDE EFFECTS

Major cyclophosphamide side effects are listed in Table 4-11. The reversible reactions occur in most treated patients but appear to be less frequent with high-dose parenteral pulses. The gastrointestinal symptoms often can be managed successfully with symptomatic therapy.

The oncogenicity of cyclophosphamide is not well established in rheumatic disease patients. Sterility resulting from the drug may or may not be reversible, and this must be made clear to men or women of child-bearing age. One of the most dreaded complications of cyclophosphamide therapy is hemorrhagic cystitis, which may occur less often with parenteral than with oral routes of administration but has been reported in up to 30% of patients receiving the drug. In either event vigorous hydration is recommended to dilute the toxic metabolites in the urinary bladder. Microscopic hematuria may be a herald of the fully developed syndrome. Although the cystitis itself is usually reversible on stopping therapy, bladder fibrosis and carcinoma have been reported as sequelae. Cyclophosphamide may predispose to infection in the absence of significant leukopenia, and a serious infection indicates at least a temporary interruption of therapy. Most reported cases of myocarditis and interstitial pulmonary fibrosis have occurred in patients receiving the drug for malignancy.

INFORMED CONSENT AND EXPENSE

Most of the rheumatic conditions for which cyclophosphamide might be indicated are sufficiently serious or life threatening to justify the use of a toxic and technically experimental agent, but informed consent for its use from the patient is essential. Not only should potential recipients be aware of its side effects and effects on reproductive function, they should also be prepared to report any symptoms suggesting serious toxicity; these symptoms include fever, sore throat, abnormal bleeding, dysuria, cough, and dyspnea.

Because of the nature of the conditions for which it is used, expense of cyclophosphamide therapy is seldom a major consideration. When used as a slow-acting agent in RA, the frequent laboratory monitoring required and the necessity of reacting to the frequent side effects make cyclophosphamide one of the more expensive of the slow-acting therapies.

Table 4-10. Cyclophosphamide use in rheumatic diseases

Disease and manifestation	Dose/route	Duration of therapy	Expected outcome	Comment
Active RA resistant to other slow-acting drugs	<1/mg/kg to >2 mg/kg PO	Limited by toxicity; less than 1 year	Moderate to marked improvement. Healing of bone erosions	Documented in controlled clinical trials. Too toxic for routine use. Low dose may be as effective as high dose.
Rheumatoid vasculitis and other severe extra-articular complications	Variable, usually about 2 mg/kg PO or as tolerated	Until recovery	Mostly satisfactory responses. Healing of vasculitis. Increased survival?	Anecdotal reports
Systemic lupus erythematosus with diffuse proliferative nephritis	500–1000 mg/m² IV every 1–3 months	For about 8 months after clinical response	Superior to other immunosuppressive programs in reducing risk of end-stage renal disease with fewer side effects	Documented in one controlled study. Numerous dosing variations being used; often the same dose monthly for 6 months

Systemic lupus erythematosus with severe vasculitis, CNS disease, or other life-threatening manifestations.	IV protocol above or about 2 mg/kg PO or as tolerated	Until recovery from the manifestations being treated	Recovery or improvement or survival	Anecdotal reports or small series
Polyarteritis and variants	About 2 mg/kg PO or as tolerated	Months to years after complete remission; total duration not established	Complete remission if treated early	Anecdotal reports and one uncontrolled trial; one negative trial
Wegener's granulomatosis	About 2 mg/kg/day PO	For at least several months, perhaps a year, after complete remission	Complete remission with no future recurrences —?cure	No controlled trials, but a large clinical experience supports this drug as the treatment of choice
Mixed cryoglobulinemia with diffuse proliferative nephritis	About 2 mg/kg/day PO	Months after complete remission	Complete remission	Anecdotal reports

Table 4-11. Major cyclophosphamide side effects

Potentially reversible or responsive to dose adjustment
  Bone marrow depression
    Leukopenia
    Thrombocytopenia
    Pancytopenia
  Gastrointestinal symptoms
    Nausea and vomiting
    Diarrhea
    Abdominal discomfort
  Alopecia
Potentially irreversible
  Carcinogenesis
  Sterility
  Hemorrhagic cystitis
  Predisposition to infections
  Myocarditis
  Interstitial pulmonary fibrosis

Other Immunoregulatory Agents

Numerous other drugs known to affect the immune system have been reported to be effective in RA and other rheumatic diseases. The list is too long to discuss all of them here, but three will be mentioned, with emphasis on cyclosporin, which may hold more promise than most others. None of these agents is FDA approved for use in any rheumatic disease.

Chlorambucil

Another alkylating agent, chlorambucil (see also under Cyclophosphamide), has been used as an alternative to cyclophosphamide, but it is generally regarded as an inferior drug for most rheumatic conditions; however, it is probably the most widely used immunosuppressive agent worldwide for Beçhet's disease, especially when uveitis is a major clinical problem. The dose usually employed is in the range of 0.1–0.2 mg/kg/day orally. Side effects are similar to those from cyclophosphamide except hemorrhagic cystitis appears not to occur. Its oncogenicity is highly significant; a marked increase in the incidence of leukemia and other malignancies has been reported with its use.

Levamisole

Levamisole was recently made available in this country for the sole indication of adjuvant therapy (with fluorouracil) for Dukes' stage C colon cancer. It is available in 50-mg tablets as Ergamisol. The drug had previously been marketed in Europe and elsewhere as a nematocidal agent. It potentiates both the inflammatory and the immune response, especially the latter. Through some interesting and circuitous reasoning, it was tried in patients with RA in the 1970s and found to be effective. Subsequent controlled clinical trials supported its efficacy as a slow-acting agent when doses of about 150 mg/day orally were used. For a while it appeared as if the drug would be FDA approved and marketed in this country for RA, but too many reports of serious granulocytopenia lead to its being abandoned. Since its actions are relatively unique, levamisole, or some analog of it, may be heard from again, however.

Cyclosporin

Cyclosporin is a fungal metabolite with highly selective immunosuppressive properties; it produces no hematopoietic suppression. The drug appears to act preferentially on proliferating T-lymphocytes and reduces IL-2 production and the cytokine cascade dependent on IL-2 (see Chapter 3 for details on interleukins). It may also have inhibitory effects on antigen-processing cells. Cyclosporin accumulates in cells through intracellular binding to cyclophilin, which is closely related, or identical, to an isomerase involved in folding of regulatory proteins. Cyclosporin is now widely used as the immunosuppressive agent of choice in renal and other transplant recipients.

The major side effect of the drug is nephrotoxicity, which develops in up to one-third of organ transplant recipients. Hepatotoxicity, hirsutism, tremors, gum hyperplasia, muscle cramps, paresthesias, and seizures also occur with its use.

Usually with doses in the range of 5–8 mg/kg/day, the drug has been found to be effective in controlled trials as a slow-acting agent in refractory RA; however, side effects, particularly nephrotoxicity, have been a significant problem. The role of cyclosporin in RA is yet to be defined, but currently there appears to be widespread enthusiasm for its investigation. More anecdotal reports have also suggested that the drug may benefit a number of other rheumatic and autoimmune diseases, including chronic active hepatitis, sarcoidosis, and inflammatory bowel disease.

Cyclosporin is marketed as Sandimmune in an oral solution containing 100 mg/ml. It is also available in a parenteral preparation for intravenous use, but this route may be more toxic than the oral one.

Choosing a SAARD in RA

Relative advantages and disadvantages of the approved slow-acting drugs and sulfasalazine are summarized in Table 4-12. Once a decision to begin slow-acting drug therapy has been made, a number of factors might influence the decision to choose one of these agents over the others for the initial trial. These factors include efficacy,

Table 4-12. Relative advantages and disadvantages of the approved slow-acting agents and sulfasalazine in RA

Agent	Relative effectiveness	Relative toxicity	Cumulative toxicity	Time to onset of action (months)	Toxicity/monitoring	Cost for 6 months ($)	Annual mainten-ance costs ($)
Parenteral gold	High; about 70% initial response rate	High; 10–15% early withdrawal rate	None significant	3–6	CBC and urinalysis before each 20 initial injections (weekly); then every other injection	1408	438
Oral gold (auranofin)	Low; about 40–50% initial response rate	Low; but up to 10% early withdrawal rate	None significant	3–6	CBC and urinalysis once a month indefinitely	500	1000
D-penicilla-mine	High; about 70% initial response rate at doses >750 mg/day	Very high; up to 40% withdrawal rate in first year	None significant	4–12 depending on dosage schedule	CBC and urinalysis every 3–4 weeks indefinitely (perhaps every 2 weeks for first few months)	636 — varies with dose	1356 — varies with dose
Azathioprine	High; about 70% initial response rate	Low-medium; about 10% early withdrawal rate	Oncogenicity not established in RA	3–9 depending on dosage schedule	CBC once a month and liver tests every 3 months indefinitely	609 — varies with dose	1352 — varies with dose

Hydroxy-chloroquine	Low; perhaps 40–50% initial response rate	Very low; <10% early withdrawal rate	3–6	Likelihood of retinopathy may increase with duration of therapy	Ophthalmologic evaluation before treatment and every 6 months indefinitely	524	524
Methotrexate	Very high; perhaps as high as 90% initial response rate	Medium–high; up to 30% initial withdrawal rate (but can be lowered with precautions)	1–2	Risk for hepatic cirrhosis not clearly established	CBC every 2–4 weeks; liver tests every 2–3 months indefinitely	270	529—varies widely with dose and route of administration
Sulfasalazine	Low; perhaps 50% initial response rate	Low; but early withdrawal rates reported as high as 25%	3–6	None recognized	CBC monthly initially; then every 2 months; periodic liver tests	402	1098—varies widely with dose and route of administration

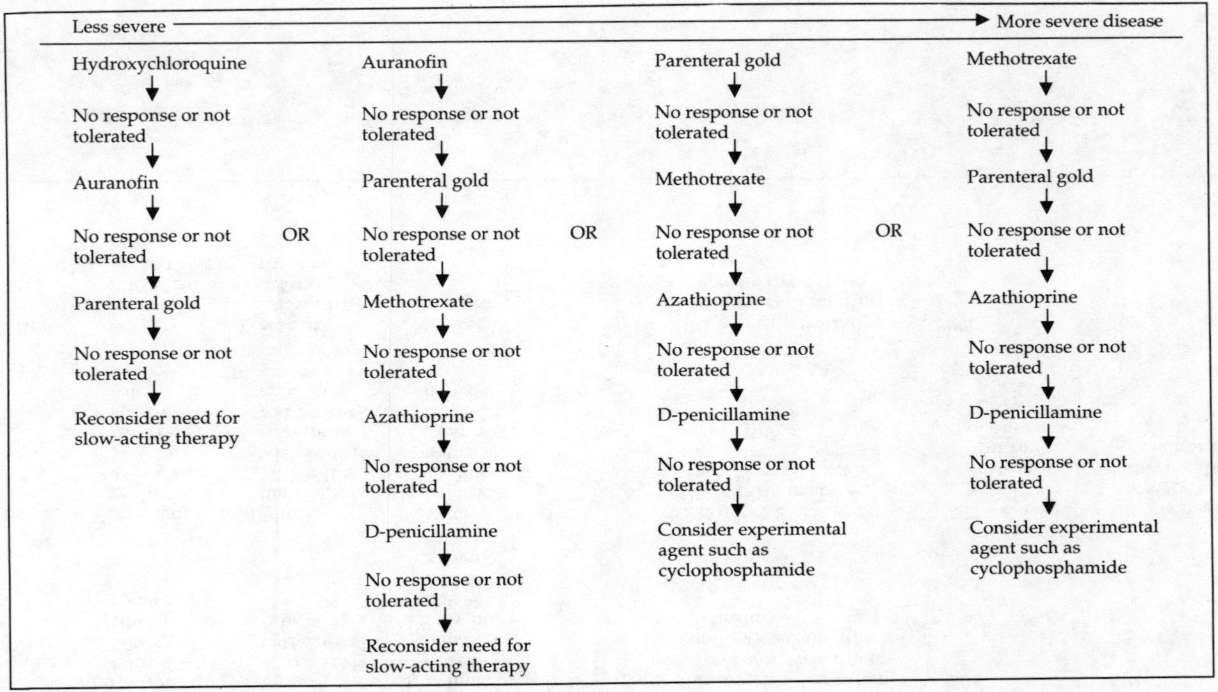

Fig. 4-10. Some possible sequences of slow-acting drug therapy in RA.

Less severe → More severe disease

Hydroxychloroquine → No response or not tolerated → **Auranofin** → No response or not tolerated → **Parenteral gold** → No response or not tolerated → **Reconsider need for slow-acting therapy**

OR

Auranofin → No response or not tolerated → **Parenteral gold** → No response or not tolerated → **Methotrexate** → No response or not tolerated → **Azathioprine** → No response or not tolerated → **D-penicillamine** → No response or not tolerated → **Reconsider need for slow-acting therapy**

OR

Parenteral gold → No response or not tolerated → **Methotrexate** → No response or not tolerated → **Azathioprine** → No response or not tolerated → **D-penicillamine** → No response or not tolerated → **Consider experimental agent such as cyclophosphamide**

OR

Methotrexate → No response or not tolerated → **Parenteral gold** → No response or not tolerated → **Azathioprine** → No response or not tolerated → **D-penicillamine** → No response or not tolerated → **Consider experimental agent such as cyclophosphamide**

safety, convenience, expense, and experience of the prescribing physician. Although a severe, rapidly progressive disease might favor the choice of one of the more effective agents, and equivocal indications for slow-acting therapy might favor the choice of one of the less toxic ones, there is no right or wrong decision. It is largely a matter of opinion. Unless the disease is very aggressive, many American rheumatologists will use auranofin or HCQ initially, opting for safety over efficacy. For the same reasons, sulfasalazine is widely used as the first slow-acting agent in Europe. Because of its obvious appeal, MTX is sometimes used initially, and that practice is currently being debated. Based on years of experience, other rheumatologists continue to prescribe parenteral gold first. Long-term safety is an important consideration that favors the initial use of one of the gold compounds.

Because of its efficacy and rapid onset of action, MTX may have become the most widely used second agent in this country after failure of one of the less toxic ones, but, again, long-term safety could suggest a trial of parenteral gold prior to resorting to MTX, considering the possibility of its cumulative hepatotoxicity. When MTX fails or is not tolerated, D-penicillamine and azathioprine continue to be available, though concerns over the potential oncogenicity of azathioprine limit its usefulness in some opinions, and D-penicillamine is clearly a difficult and expensive drug to work with. A number of possible sequences are illustrated in Fig. 4-10.

Several clinical trials have attempted to evaluate the efficacy and safety of combinations of two slow-acting agents used simultaneously. Typically combinations have been chosen on the basis of distinctly different toxicity profiles. The addition of HCQ to other more effective slow-acting agents does not clearly result in enhanced benefits though enhanced toxicity has not been a problem. There is tentative evidence, however, that the addition of sulfasalazine to an auranofin program or to a course of one of the more effective agents may result in added benefits without increasing toxicity, though this practice remains experimental. Even if safety and enhanced efficacy of combinations of slow-acting agents are clearly documented, expense will likely limit their use; however, a recent survey of rheumatologists indicated that about half were using some type of combination slow-acting therapy.

Bibliography

PARENTERAL GOLD

Aaron, S., Davis, P., and Percy, J. Neutropenia occurring during the course of chrysotherapy: A review of 25 cases. *J. Rheumatol.* 12:897–899, 1985.

Adachi, J. D., et al. Gold induced thrombocytopenia: 12 cases and a review of the literature. *Semin. Arthritis Rheum.* 16:287–293, 1987.

Clark, P., et al. Meta-analysis of injectable gold in rheumatoid arthritis. *J. Rheumatol.* 16:442–447, 1989.

Empire Rheumatism Council. Gold therapy in rheumatoid arthritis. *Ann. Rheum. Dis.* 20:315–334, 1961.

Furst, D. E., et al. A double-blind trial of high versus convential dosages of gold salts for rheumatoid arthritis. *Arthritis Rheum.* 20:1473–1480, 1977.

Gibbons, R. B. Complications of chrysotherapy. *Arch. Intern. Med.* 139:343–346, 1979.

Gordon, D. A. Gold Compounds. In W. N. Kelley et al. (eds.), *Textbook of Rheumatology* (3rd ed.). Philadelphia: Saunders, 1989. Pp. 804–823.

Graham, C. G., and Dale, M. M. The activation of gold complexes by cyanide produced by polymorphonuclear leukocytes II: Evidence for the formation and biologic activity of aurocyanide. *Biochem. Pharmacol.* 39:1697–1702, 1990.

Hall, C. L., et al. The natural course of gold nephropathy: long term study of 21 patients. *Br. Med. J.* 295:745–748, 1987.

Lockie, L. M., and Smith, D. M. Forty-seven years experience with gold therapy in 1,019 rheumatoid arthritis patients. *Semin. Arthritis Rheum.* 14:238–246, 1985.

Yan, A., and Davis, P. Gold induced marrow suppression: A review of 10 cases. *J. Rheumatol.* 17:47–51, 1990.

AURANOFIN

Bombardier, C., et al. Auranofin therapy and quality of life in patients with rheumatoid arthritis. *Am. J. Med.* 81:565–578, 1986.

Capell, H. A., Lewis, D., and Carey, J. A three year follow up of patients allocated to placebo, or oral or injectable gold therapy for rheumatoid arthritis. *Ann. Rheum. Dis.* 45:705–711, 1986.

Champion, G. D., et al. Dose response studies and longterm evaluation of auranofin in rheumatoid arthritis. *J. Rheumatol.* 15:28–34, 1988.

Davis, P., et al. One-year comparative study of gold sodium thiomalate and auranofin in the treatment of rheumatoid arthritis. *J. Rheumatol.* 12:60–67, 1985.

Herlin, T., et al. Effect of auranofin on eicosanoids and protein kinase in human neutrophils. *Agents Actions* 28:121–129, 1989.

Snyder, R. M., Mirabelli, C. K., and Crooke, S. T. The cellular pharmacology of auranofin. *Semin. Arthritis Rheum.* 17:71–80, 1987.

Wallin, B. A., et al. Incidence and management of diarrhea during longterm auranofin therapy. *J. Rheumatol.* 15:1755–1758, 1988.

Ward, J. R., et al. Comparison of auranofin, gold sodium thiomalate, and placebo in the treatment of rheumatoid arthritis. *Arthritis Rheum.* 26:1303–1315, 1983.

Williams, H. J., et al. One-year experience in patients treated with auranofin following completion of a parallel, controlled trial comparing auranofin, gold sodium thiomalate, and placebo. *Arthritis Rheum.* 31:9–14, 1988.

D-PENICILLAMINE

Cooperative Systematic Studies of Rheumatic Disease Group. Toxicity of longterm low dose D-penicillamine therapy in rheumatoid arthritis. *J. Rheumatol.* 14:67–73, 1987.

Hall, C. L., et al. Natural course of penicillamine nephropathy: a long term study of 33 patients. *Br. Med. J.* 296:1083–1086, 1988.

Howard-Lock, H. E., et al. D-penicillamine: Chemistry and clinical use in rheumatic disease. *Semin. Arthritis Rheum.* 15:261–281, 1986.

Jaffe, I. A. Induction of auto-immune syndromes by penicillamine therapy in rheumatoid arthritis and other diseases. *Springer Semin. Immunopathol.* 4:193–207, 1981.

Kean, W. F., et al. Prior gold therapy does not influence the adverse effects of D-penicillamine in rheumatoid arthritis. *Arthritis Rheum.* 25:917–922, 1982.

Muijsers, A. O., et al. D-penicillamine in patients with rheumatoid arthritis. *Arthritis Rheum.* 27:1362–1369, 1984.

Thomas, M. H., et al. Gold vs D-penicillamine double blind study and followup. *J. Rheumatol.* 11:764–767, 1984.

Williams, H. J., et al. Low-dose D-penicillamine therapy in rheumatoid arthritis. *Arthritis Rheum.* 26:581–592, 1983.

AZATHIOPRINE

Paulus, H. E., et al. Azathioprine versus D-penicillamine in rheumatoid arthritis patients who have been treated unsuccessfully with gold. *Arthritis Rheum.* 27:721–727, 1984.

Silman, A. J., et al. Lymphoproliferative cancer and other malignancy in patients with rheumatoid arthritis treated with azathioprine: a 20 year follow up study. *Ann. Rheum. Dis.* 47:988–992, 1988.

Singh, G., et al. Toxic effects of azathioprine in rheumatoid arthritis. *Arthritis Rheum.* 32:837–843, 1989.

Urowitz, M. B., et al. Azathioprine in rheumatoid arthritis: A double-blind study comparing full dose to half dose. *J. Rheumatol.* 1:274–281, 1974.

Voogd, C. E. Azathioprine, a genotoxic agent to be considered nongenotoxic in man. *Mutat. Res.* 221:133–152, 1989.

ANTIMALARIALS

Bellany, N., and Brooks, P. M. Current practice in antimalarial drug prescribing in rheumatoid arthritis. *J. Rheumatol.* 13:551–555, 1986.

Bunch, T. W., et al. Controlled trial of hydroxychloroquine and D-penicillamine singly and in combination in the treatment of rheumatoid arthritis. *Arthritis Rheum.* 27:267–276, 1984.

The Canadian Hydroxychloroquine Study Group. A randomized study of the effect of withdrawing hydroxychloroquine sulfate in systemic lupus erythematosus. *N. Engl. J. Med.* 324:150–154, 1991.

Maksymowych, W., and Russell, A. S. Antimalarials in rheumatology: Efficacy and safety. *Semin. Arthritis Rheum.* 16:206–221, 1987.

Pavelka, K., Jr., et al. Hydroxychloroquine sulphate in the treatment of rheumatoid arthritis: a double-blind comparison of two dose regimens. *Ann. Rheum. Dis.* 48:542–546, 1989.

Rynes, R. I. Antimalarial Drugs. In W. N. Kelley et al. (eds.), *Textbook of Rheumatology* (3rd ed.). Philadelphia. Saunders, 1989. Pp. 792–803.

Titus, E. O. Recent developments in the understanding of the pharmacokinetics and mechanism of action of chloroquine. *Ther. Drug Monit.* 11:369–379, 1989.

METHOTREXATE

Alarcon, G. S., Tracy, I. C., and Blackburn, W. D., Jr. Methotrexate in rheumatoid arthritis. *Arthritis Rheum.* 32:671–676, 1989.

Carson, C. W., et al. Pulmonary disease during the treatment of rheumatoid arthritis with low-dose pulse methotrexate. *Semin. Arthritis Rheum.* 16:186–195, 1987.

Hamdy, H., et al. Low-dose methotrexate compared with azathioprine in the treatment of rheumatoid arthritis. *Arthritis Rheum.* 30:361–367, 1987.

Kremer, J. M., and Kaye, G. I. Electron microscopic analysis of sequential liver biopsy samples from patients with rheumatoid arthritis. *Arthritis Rheum.* 32:1202–1213, 1989.

Kremer, J. M., and Lee, J. K. A long-term prospective study of the use of methotrexate in rheumatoid arthritis. *Arthritis Rheum.* 31:577–584, 1988.

Kremer, J. M., Lee, R. G., and Tolman, K. G. Liver histology in rheumatoid arthritis patients receiving long-term methotrexate therapy. *Arthritis Rheum.* 32:121–127, 1989.

Morgan, S. L., et al. The effect of folic acid supplementation on the toxicity of low-dose methotrexate in patients with rheumatoid arthritis. *Arthritis Rheum.* 33:9–18, 1990.

Nordstrom, D. M., et al. Pulse methotrexate therapy in rheumatoid arthritis. *Ann. Intern. Med.* 107:797–801, 1987.

Olsen, N. J., Callahan, L. F., and Pincus, T. Immunologic studies of rheumatoid arthritis patients treated with methotrexate. *Arthritis Rheum.* 30:481–488, 1987.

Tugwell, P., Bennett, K., and Gent, M. Methotrexate in rheumatoid arthritis. *Ann. Intern. Med.* 107:358–366, 1987.

Weinblatt, M. E., et al. Low-dose methotrexate compared with auranofin in adult rheumatoid arthritis. *Arthritis Rheum.* 33:330–338, 1990.

Williams, H. J., et al. Comparison of low-dose oral pulse methotrexate and placebo in the treatment of rheumatoid arthritis. *Arthritis Rheum.* 28:721–730, 1985.

SULFASALAZINE

Amos, R. S., et al. Sulphasalazine for rheumatoid arthritis: toxicity in 774 patients monitored for one to 11 years. *Br. Med. J.* 293:420–423, 1986.

Comer, S. S., and Jasin, H. E. In vitro immunomodulatory effects of sulfasalazine and its metabolites. *J. Rheumatol.* 15:580–586, 1988.

Dawes, P. T., et al. Improving the response to gold or D-penicillamine by addition of sulphasalazine. A pilot study in 25 patients with rheumatoid arthritis. *Clin. Exp. Rheumatol.* 5:151–153, 1987.

Neumann, V. C., et al. A study to determine the active moiety of sulphasalazine in rheumatoid arthritis. *J. Rheumatol.* 13:285–287, 1986.

Nuver-Zwart, I. H., et al. A double blind comparative study of sulphasalazine and hydroxychloroquine in rheumatoid arthritis: evidence of an earlier effect of sulphasalazine. *Ann. Rheum. Dis.* 48:389–395, 1989.

Pinals, R. S. Sulfasalazine in the rheumatic disease. *Semin. Arthritis Rheum.* 17:246–259, 1988.

Symmons, D. P., et al. Sulfasalazine treatment and lymphocyte function in patients with rheumatoid arthritis. *J. Rheumatol.* 15:575–579, 1988.

Williams, H. J., et al. A controlled trial comparing sulfasalazine, gold sodium thiomalate, and placebo in rheumatoid arthritis. *Arthritis Rheum.* 31:702–713, 1988.

OTHER IMMUNOREGULATORY AGENTS AND OVERVIEWS

Baltus, J. A. M., et al. The occurrence of malignancies in patients with rheumatoid arthritis treated with cyclophosphamide: a controlled retrospective follow-up. *Ann. Rheum. Dis.* 42:368–373, 1983.

Clements, P. J., and Davis, J. Cytotoxic drugs: their clinical application to the rheumatic diseases. *Semin. Arthritis Rheum.* 15:231–254, 1986.

Cooperating Clinics Committee of the American Rheumatism Association. A controlled trial of cyclophosphamide in rheumatoid arthritis. *N. Engl. J. Med.* 283:883–889, 1970.

Dougados, M., Awada, H., and Amor, B. Cyclosporin in rheumatoid arthritis: a double blind, placebo controlled study in 52 patients. *Ann. Rheum. Dis.* 47:127–133, 1988.

Fauci, A. S., et al. Immunomodulators in clinical medicine. *Ann. Intern. Med.* 106:421–433, 1987.

Fox, D. A., and McCune, W. J. Immunologic and Clinical Effects of Cytotoxic Drugs Used in the Treatment of Rheumatoid Arthritis and Systemic Lupus Erythematosus. In J. M. Cruse and R. E. Lewis Jr (eds.), *Therapy of Autoimmune Diseases* (Vol. 7). Basel: Karger, 1989. Pp. 20–78.

Kovarsky, J. Clinical pharmacology and toxicology of cyclophosphamide: emphasis on use in rheumatic diseases. *Semin. Arthritis Rheum.* 12:359–372, 1983.

Lipsky, P. E. Mechanisms of action of slow-acting drugs in rheumatoid arthritis. *Clin. Exp. Rheumatol.* 7(S/3):177–180, 1989.

McCune, W. J., and Bayliss, G. E. Immunosuppressive drug therapy. *Curr. Opinion Rheumatol.* 1:80–88, 1989.

Multicentre Study Group. Levamisole in rheumatoid arthritis. *Ann. Rheum. Dis.* 41:159–163, 1982.

Shepard, V. L. Intracellular pathways and mechanisms of sorting in receptor-mediated endocytosis. *TIPS* 10:458–462, 1989.

St. Georgiev, V. Immunomodulatory activity of small peptides. *TIPS* 11:373–378, 1990.

Tsokos, G. C. Immunomodulatory treatment in patients with rheumatic diseases: mechanisms of action. *Semin. Arthritis Rheum.* 17:24–38, 1987.

Tugwell, P., et al. Low-dose cyclosporin versus placebo in patients with rheumatoid arthritis. *Lancet* 335:1051–1055, 1990.

5

Drugs Used in the Treatment of Gout and Pseudogout

Included in this chapter is a group of agents that share a role in the management of the crystalline-induced arthropathies. Three distinctively different pharmacologic actions are involved: treatment of acute attacks of crystalline-induced synovitis, prevention of recurring attacks of synovitis, and normalizing the serum uric acid in order to mobilize tissue urate deposits and prevent their further accumulation. Colchicine specifically accomplishes the first two actions and allopurinol and the uricosuric drugs accomplish the latter one. Colchicine has no effect on serum uric acid itself, but it does have a number of actions that make it useful in the management of diseases other than the crystalline-induced arthropathies. This drug is included in this section only because it does not seem to fit in any better elsewhere.

The Concept of Crystalline-Induced Disease

In order to understand the actions and clinical indications for these agents, it is necessary to understand the concept of crystalline-induced disease. Although several crystals have been shown to be or are thought to be pathogenic in humans, specific therapy has been documented to be effective for the consequences of only two: monosodium urate (or uric acid) and calcium pyrophosphate dihydrate (CPPD). Uric acid crystal deposition results in the disease called **gout**, and CPPD crystal deposition results in somewhat of a semantic problem. **CPPD deposition disease** is an acceptable term but is not often used. Most chondrocalcinosis (by joint radiographs) is due to CPPD deposition, and this term is often used synonymously with CPPD deposition disease. An acute attack of arthritis associated with this disease is called **pseudogout**, another term often used synonymously with chondrocalcinosis or CPPD deposition disease. In the following discussion, pseudogout will be used to refer only to the acute arthritis.

Urate deposition disease or gout results from sustained hyperuricemia, which is usually primary or idiopathic, but may be secondary to urate overproduction from some known cause or due to urate underexcretion secondary to some identifiable drug or toxin (Table 5-1). After years of a persisting supersaturated plasma uric acid level, crystalline deposits develop in synovial structures (joint lining, bursae, tendon sheaths) and in the kidney (interstitially or in the form of renal stones). When these deposits become clinically apparent on physical examination or by joint radiographs, they are called **tophi**. In some patients (but not all) with synovial urate crystalline

Table 5-1. Factors that cause hyperuricemia

Factor	Mechanism	Comments
Aspirin, NSAIDs, low doses	Decreased secretion	High doses uricosuric
Thiazide (loop) diuretics	Decreased secretion, competition	
Ethambutol	Decreased secretion	Probenecid responsive
Pyrazinamide	Decreased secretion	**Not** responsive to probenecid; blocked by acetylsalicylic acid, 5-NH$_2$-salicylate
6-MP, azathioprine, cytotoxic agents, radiation, etc.	Increased production	Blocked by allopurinol
Lead poisoning	Renal tubular damage	
Sickle cell anemia	Increased production	
Chronic alcoholism	Increased production	Decreased excretion with high blood levels
Organic acidoses	Decreased secretion	Occurs with ketosis alone

deposits, discrete attacks of acute arthritis, bursitis, or less often tenosynovitis may begin to occur relatively late in the course of the hyperuricemia; this phenomenon is usually referred to as **articular gout**. The attacks are often precipitated by relatively sudden changes (up or down) in serum urate levels. After articular gout becomes clinically apparent, the patient is at increased risk for clinically apparent renal gout and for tophaceous joint destruction, perhaps the most undesirable outcome in patients with the disease. In untreated gout, the acute attacks of arthritis tend to become more frequent and more polyarticular with time, and they may be disabling to some patients, even in the absence of joint destruction.

Uric acid is freely filtered by the renal glomerulus, almost completely reabsorbed in the more proximal part of the tubule, and then secreted in the more distal part of the tubule. A number of drugs and toxins may interfere with reabsorption or secretion or sometimes both. Obviously, blocking reabsorption increases urate excretion and lowers serum uric levels, whereas blocking secretion has the opposite effect. Under certain circumstances (usually tumor lysis), urate production may be so massive as to completely overwhelm the tubular reabsorptive mechanisms, resulting in extraordinarily high urate concentrations in the tubular filtrate. Consequently urate precipitation may occur in the tubule, leading to acute tubular necrosis. This phenomenon is usually not considered part of the spectrum of gout, but it represents the only other recognized important clinical consequence of hyperuricemia.

Unlike gout, CPPD deposition has no recognized underlying biochemical defect, though it is associated with diseases, such as hyperparathyroidism and hemachromatosis, that do. Furthermore, unlike gout, CPPD crystals tend to deposit only in joint cartilages, initially fibrocartilage and later hyalin cartilage. The clinical consequences are osteoarthritis (which cannot be prevented) and pseudogout (which can be both prevented and treated). Consequently the pharmacology of CPPD deposition disease will be much simpler than the pharmacology of gout, and the pharmacologic prevention and treatment of pseudogout are virtually identical to the prevention and treatment of acute articular gout.

Hyperuricemia and the Pathogenesis of Gout

As presented earlier in this chapter, the ultimate predisposing factor to deposition of uric acid in/on the lining of joint spaces is hyperuricemia. It is essential to an adequate presentation of the mechanisms of effect of several drugs used in the management of gout (Fig. 5-1) that formation of uric acid as well as its disposition in the body are understood; therefore, both aspects are presented briefly here. Alterations in formation or excretion or both of uric acid that may contribute to hyperuricemia are covered briefly also. A partial listing of drug agents and conditions known to produce hyperuricemia is provided in Table 5-1.

FORMATION OF URIC ACID

Uric acid is an end product of purine metabolism in humans (see Fig. 5-5, under allopurinol). Uric acid is not further converted and is excreted (daily total usually < 1 gm). Several chemical characteristics of uric acid are worthy of note. Uric acid is quite insoluble and its solubility is markedly affected by pH. The relevance of the former observation is that, at physiologic pH, uric acid concentrations in excess of 7 mg% can result in crystal formation/deposition. The latter observation relates to the fact that uric acid is a weak organic acid with a pK_a of 5.5: At pH below its pK_a, the acid form, which is **very** insoluble, predominates and crystallization becomes even more probable. The converse is also true, i.e., as pH exceeds 5.5, the urate (sodium salt) form becomes increasingly predominant and solubility increases. This is **not** to say that sodium urate is very soluble, only more soluble than the free acid. It should be noted that a small amount of urate binding to plasma proteins occurs and may result in some increase in urate solubility. Displacement of this small fraction could disturb a precarious solubility balance.

The statement that uric acid is an end product of purine metabolism must be viewed in light of the fact that, unlike its immediate precursors, hypoxanthine and xanthine, uric acid cannot be recycled back to purines (adenosine monophosphate [AMP], guanosine monophosphate [GMP], respectively) and thus participate in nucleic acid synthesis, via salvage pathways. Changes in activity of the salvage pathway may in fact contribute to hyperuricemia. For example, the enzyme hypoxanthine-guanine phosphoribosyltransferase (HGPRT), a main participant in salvage, is deficient in the Lesch-Nyhan syndrome, which has an associated hyperuricemia. Apparently, excess xanthine and hypoxanthine are converted to uric acid. Deficiencies

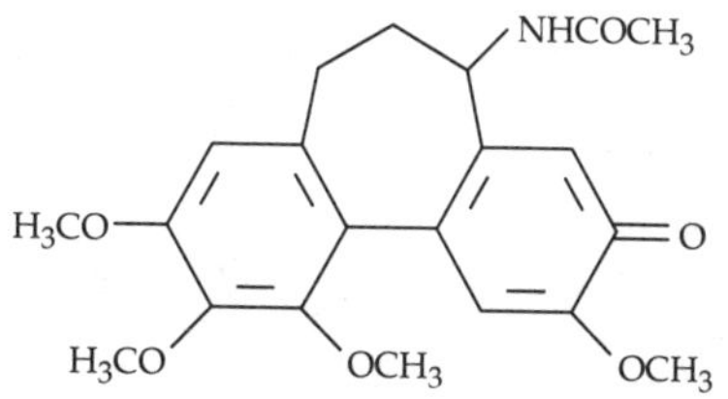

Colchicine

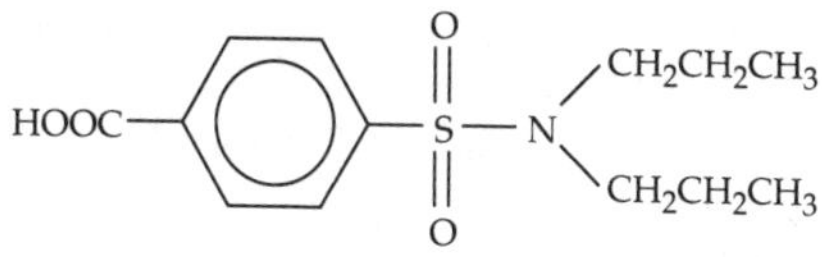

Probenecid

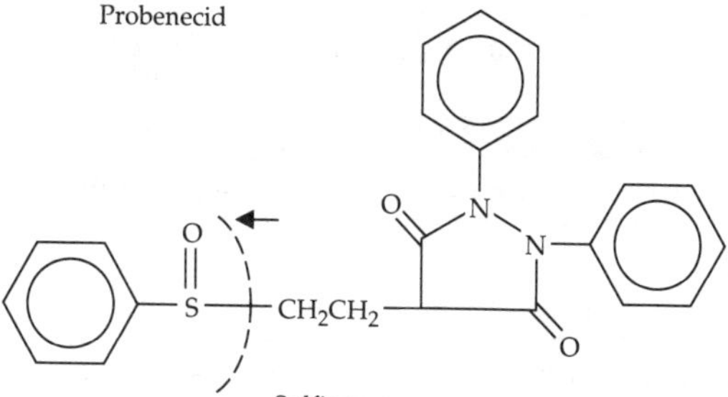

Sulfinpyrazone

$(CH_3CH_2 \dashv\!\!-$, phenylbutazone)

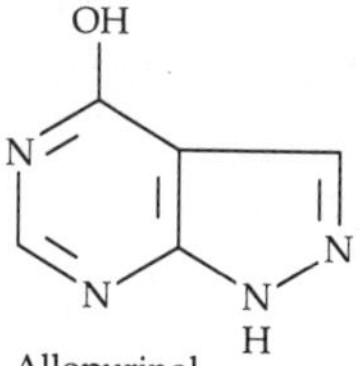

Allopurinol

Fig. 5-1. Structures of various drugs used in the management of gout. (See also Fig. 5-5.)

of HGPRT unrelated to Lesch-Nyhan have been identified. Alterations in other enzymes impinging on uric acid production have also been suggested as causative or permissive to hyperuricemia and gout.

In addition to metabolic overproduction due to enzyme changes, oversupply of purines for degradation can also cause overproduction. Oversupply **may** be a dietary consideration under some conditions (chronic renal crystallization/stone formation). Large-scale cellular disruption, initiated by any of several possible circumstances, is a more likely and common cause, however. The circumstances usually relate to malignancy, even untreated, but more so to malignancy treated by radiation or cytotoxic agents resulting in the death of large numbers of cells.

EXCRETION OF URIC ACID

Uric acid, as most weak organic acids, is excreted primarily via the kidney. Several processes contribute to the overall renal dynamics of uric acid. Because it is a relatively small molecule, uric acid/urate is freely filtered in the glomeruli. It has been suggested that decreased renal blood flow (atherosclerotic or vasoconstrictive/hypertension in origin) can decrease filtration and thus predispose to hyperuricemia in some instances.

Filtered urate is very efficiently reabsorbed, primarily in the proximal tubule, but also in more distal segments. The process of reabsorption is carrier mediated (facilitated transport) and thus of limited, albeit high, capacity. Interference with reabsorption causes uric acid to remain in the tubules (uricosuria) and can lead to decreased levels in blood. In instances wherein the filtered amounts are extremely high (e.g., malignancy), the ceiling on reabsorption may be exceeded, and very high uric acid concentrations in tubular fluid/urine may persist. The latter situation, and occasionally simple hyperuricemia, can lead to crystallization in the tubules, especially if pH is low.

Uric acid is a substrate for the proximal tubular weak organic acid (organic anion) secretory carrier. A significant amount of uric acid can be added to tubular fluid via this route. Impaired function of the secretory mechanism (e.g., via competition by other weak organic acids including drugs) can (further) increase blood levels of uric acid, especially if reabsorption is unimpaired.

With all renal processes operative without impairment or interference, net excretion (filtration − reabsorption + secretion) is about 10% of the secreted load, which is equivalent to slightly less than 5% of the filtered load. The processes involved in renal uric acid dynamics are summarized in Fig. 5-2.

MECHANISMS AND MEDIATORS OF URIC ACID CRYSTAL-INDUCED INFLAMMATION

The inflammation of acute gout, even without treatment, is relatively short term and will usually resolve in several days to no more than several weeks without intervention. Intervention is usually sought, however, because of the major discomfort experienced, and the event can be significantly shortened pharmacologically. The mediators involved in inflammation in gout may be a subset of those involved in more chronic inflammatory states, and the initiation is better, if not perfectly, understood. Leukocytes, specifically phagocytic leukocytes (e.g., neutrophils, monocytes/macrophages), are major contributors to establishing and maintaining the intense cycle of inflammation that is characteristic of acute gout.

Free spicules of uric acid (sodium urate) that occur in the joint space and initiate inflammation probably arise from deposits on the struc-

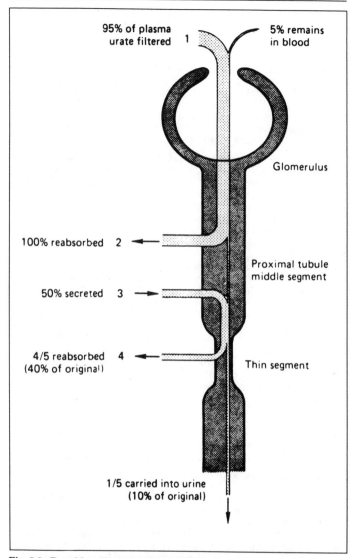

Fig. 5-2. Renal handling of uric acid. Ninety-five percent of plasma urate is filtered by the glomerulus (site 1). Urate is completely reabsorbed in the middle segment of the proximal tubule (site 2), but 50% of this is secreted by the weak acid carrier in the same portion of the nephron (site 3). Finally, of the secreted uric acid, four-fifths (40% of original) is reabsorbed at a downstream site (site 4). (Modified and reproduced, with permission, from A. Meyers, E. Jawetz, and A. Goldfien, *Review of Medical Pharmacology*, (7th ed.). East Norwalk, CT: Lange, 1980.)

tures around the space, rather than by crystallization from super-saturated fluid. The spicules per se have little effect on leukocytes (while external), but "coated" spicules rapidly activate neutrophils.

Urate spicules contact-activate Hageman factor (XII), resulting in initiation of the coagulation cascade as well as formation of kalli-krein and increased levels of bradykinin; the kinins in turn release eicosanoids. Bradykinin and the eicosanoids, and other mediators, act synergistically to cause pain and inflammatory changes, including increased vascular permeability and movement of fluid into tissue. Kallikrein also activates complement (C1, C5) and accelerates conversion of plasminogen to plasmin.

A coating of several proteins, some formed in response to the spicules themselves, rapidly occurs on spicule surfaces. The coating includes complement components as well as immunoglobulins. The latter attach to the crystals with the Fc portion left free to interact with surface receptors of leukocytes. Coated particles are phagocytosed and freed of their protein coating by lysosomal enzymes. "Clean" crystals inside the cell apparently can interact with, and elicit lysis of, cell membranes. Neutrophils activated by urate crystals thus release not only superoxide and leukotriene B_4 (LTB_4), but also proteolytic enzymes, and the original offending crystals. Release of LTB_4 prior to cell destruction acts to recruit additional cells to the area, and the cycle can continue. The inflammation cycle may be further accentuated by decreases in pH subsequent to increased populations and metabolic activity of invading leukocytes in a poorly vascularized area. The cycle continues until interrupted, naturally (e.g., crystal solubilization/redistribution, redeposition) or pharmacologically. Aspects of the crystal-inflammation cycle are summarized in Fig. 5-3. Specific pharmacologic agents that interfere with formation of uric acid (allopurinol), increase its excretion (probenecid, sulfinpyrazone), or interfere with its inflammatory effects (colchicine) are discussed in separate sections that follow.

Colchicine

Colchicine is the antiquity of the rheumatic disease pharmacopeia. It is an alkaloid of the autumn crocus plant (*Colchicum autumnale*), extracts of which were first used for joint symptoms in the sixth century A.D. and first clearly used for gout in the eighteenth century. Colchicine was isolated in 1920 and since then its effects on articular gout have become legendary. It is one of the few antique drugs in all of medicine that is more widely used and for more purposes today than it was a century ago. Although inhibited by lack of support on the part of the pharmaceutical industry, clinical trials in the past decade or so have begun to explore the utility of the drug in a number of diseases beyond the crystalline-induced arthropathies. For example, it appears to prevent the amyloidosis of familial Mediterranean fever and to enhance survival in the more common forms of amyloidosis seen in this country.

Colchicine is available generically in 0.5-mg and 0.6-mg tablets and in a parenteral solution (only for intravenous use) in a concentration of 0.5 mg/ml.

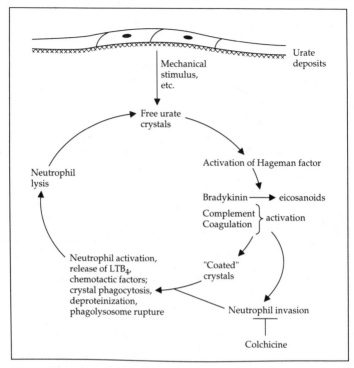

Fig. 5-3. Schematic for crystal-induced inflammatory cycle. (—, inhibits; LTB$_4$, leukotriene B$_4$.)

BASIC PHARMACOLOGY

General Properties

Colchicine is a complex, multiply methoxylated, multiringed structure (see Fig. 5-1). Despite this, it is well absorbed after oral administration. The drug distributes broadly and concentrates in several tissues, two of which are worthy of particular note: the gastrointestinal system and leukocytes. Accumulation of colchicine occurs against a concentration gradient, i.e., cells continue to increase internal levels even when external levels are lower.

Concentration in the gastrointestinal system appears to be related to the most common side effects of colchicine, i.e., cramping, diarrhea, nausea, and vomiting. Gastrointestinal effects probably result in part from decreased turnover of otherwise rapidly dividing and replenished cell populations. Oral administration increases the probability of these side effects by direct exposure. In contrast, parenteral (intravenous) administration minimizes (but does not eliminate) gastrointestinal effects, probably by limiting exposure to distribution through blood only. Colchicine concentrates in the liver and undergoes hepatic metabolism (N-deacetylation). Both free colchicine and metabolites are secreted into bile, recycled, and eventually excreted. The route of excretion thus also contributes to gastrointestinal exposure and effects. A small portion of colchicine is eliminated via the kidney, which also accumulates the drug; the fraction can increase significantly in liver dysfunction.

Colchicine accumulates in leukocytes and is avidly retained, probably due to intracellular binding to tubulin and other molecules and structures. Significant amounts of colchicine can be detected for longer than a week after a single intravenous injection. This may account for the ability of a single acute course of drug administration to effect relief. Also, leukocyte retention accounts for the recommended waiting periods between short courses of drug by this route or between oral and intravenous routes (see Clinical Indications).

Mechanism of Action

Several actions of colchicine probably contribute to its specific interruption of the inflammatory cycle in gout. The mechanism generally considered to be primary is inhibition of leukocyte movement (diapedesis). The mechanism by which this is accomplished is probably identical to the mechanism whereby colchicine inhibits cell division at metaphase: Microtubule assembly, necessary for diapedesis and for completion of cell division, is prevented by colchicine. There are also additional consequences of colchicine-altered microtubule dynamics for neutrophil function.

Colchicine may interrupt microtubule assembly through attachment to tubulin, a heterodimeric (α,β dimer) protein that is the building block of microtubules. The binding site for colchicine is probably on the α-subunit, although other (additional?) sites also have been proposed. Colchicine binding has been described as pseudoirreversible, i.e., once bound, its dissociation is very slow, such that bound and free drug are not in equilibrium. The consequences of this are that drug effect can accumulate, even at very low drug concentrations, and thus measurements of drug concentrations will not accurately depict the degree of binding that is more relevant to effect.

Subsequent to colchicine binding, drug-dimer complexes are incorporated at the growing end of a polymer. Incorporation of additional tubulin is subsequently limited due to significantly reduced affinity of the drug-containing polymer for tubulin. The guanosinetriphosphatase activity associated with the tubulin dimer is stimulated by colchicine, an effect usually associated with conformational changes that occur during addition of the dimer to a growing polymer. Thus, colchicine may not only terminate chain growth by attachment to polymers, it may also make dimers unsuitable for incorporation.

Based on comparative studies of analogs of colchicine, some of which are anti-inflammatory but do not interact with tubulin, the microtubule mechanism of action has been questioned; however, it has been suggested (but not documented) that the analogs may be converted in part to colchicine itself in vivo. The effects of analogs could thus be explained by the cumulative effect potential of even low concentrations of colchicine described previously. The microtubule assembly mechanism as sole explanation may also be questioned on the basis that other drugs that interfere with assembly and even interact at the same tubulin site as colchicine (e.g., benzimidazole antihelminthics such as mebendazole) have not been reported to have gout anti-inflammatory activity.

An alternate/additional hypothesis for mechanism of effect suggests that colchicine binds to tubulin associated with structures that regulate calcium levels in the cell (e.g., mitochondria, endoplasmic reticulum) and does so at concentrations lower than those required for interference with microtubule integrity. Since calcium promotes tubulin depolymerization and thus microtubule disassembly, such a mechanism might imply that cellular calcium levels increase in response to colchicine; calcium level changes in response to this drug have not been reported.

Effects of colchicine on other functions of neutrophils have been noted and may be related to effects on microtubules as well as to anti-inflammatory effects. For example, enzyme release and degranulation are inhibited, as is generation of LTB_4. Increased granule association with microtubules appears to be an intermediate step subsequent to cell stimulation/activation. In macrophages, treatment with colchicine specifically results in disappearance of surface receptors for tumor necrosis factor (TNF_α), suggesting the possibility that other receptors on this and other types of cells may also be regulated through microtubules. Disappearance of receptors, in conjunction with decreased release and motility limitations, may thus all contribute to colchicine's total anti-inflammatory effect.

Consequences of Use

The most common side effects produced by colchicine are gastrointestinal, as already noted. Side effects are not limited to the gut, however, and can occur in any system in the body, especially, but not exclusively, subsequent to very high doses of the drug. Because of its hepatic and renal excretion, toxicity occurs more frequently and severely in individuals with dysfunction of these organs. Dose per time limits have been developed to limit serious acute toxicity in the majority of recipients.

The explicit mechanisms for many colchicine side effects are not known; however, the rare agranulocytosis, aplastic anemia, and alopecia are most probably the result of antimitotic effects; these side effects are more likely for chronic administration. The list of possible side effects also includes several ascribable to the CNS, including decreased body temperature, respiratory depression, hypertension, and death. Death has been reported after a single 7-mg dose.

CLINICAL INDICATIONS AND DOSAGE SCHEDULES

Gout

Colchicine has no effect on serum uric acid or urate deposits; it is useful only in treating acute attacks of articular gout and in preventing recurring attacks. When used for acute attacks, the drug is much more likely to be effective when given early in the course; the response will seldom be very impressive if the joint inflammation has been present for a week or longer. Many textbooks continue to recommend oral therapy, but few experienced clinicians continue this practice. The recommended dose was usually about 1 mg q1–2 h until the attack subsided or to a total dose of 10 mg. With this approach several hours of therapy are required, and gastrointestinal side effects are extremely common and often interrupt the treatment before it has a chance to be effective. It is **not** recommended.

Instead 2 mg given intravenously over about 30 minutes is more predictably and rapidly effective with fewer side effects. A single dose is usually effective within a few hours (6–12), but an additional dose of 1 mg may be necessary later to completely alleviate the symptoms. No more than 4 mg should be given intravenously in a 24-hour period, and none should be given in any form for about a week after the initial therapy. Colchicine is very irritating if extravasation occurs, and adequate attention has to go into preventing this. Therapeutic doses of the drug, by any route, should not be used in patients with severe renal or hepatic insufficiency. The use of therapeutic colchicine as a diagnostic test for acute articular gout is much discussed. It is true that most noncrystalline arthropathies should not respond to it, but pseudogout will, and there are much better diagnostic tests (crystal identification) for gout than its response to this agent. Consequently colchicine seems to have few advantages over other drugs used for acute articular gout, and adequate doses of indomethacin (and perhaps other nonsteroidal antiinflammatory drugs [NSAIDs]) and corticosteroids are probably equally effective.

As a prophylactic agent against recurring acute articular gout, low-dose daily colchicine has been reported to reduce attack frequency by about 85%. A true prophylactic action may be unique to colchicine. Doses have usually been in the range of 0.6 mg bid, but 0.6 mg once a day may be almost as effective and might be the beginning dose. A prophylactic program is especially useful in the first few months of beginning and adjusting antihyperuricemic therapy, when attacks often occur with an increased frequency. It is best to begin prophylaxis several days prior to starting a uricosuric drug or allopurinol. In that case prophylactic oral colchicine might be started even while the attack is being treated with some other agent; it has been recommended that oral colchicine not be given for a week after completion of intravenous therapy, and it will not be needed in any event. Therapeutic and prophylactic colchicine should not be confused with each other. The doses used for prophylaxis will have no significant effect on the acute attack.

If prophylaxis is employed in patients not receiving uric acid–lowering therapy, it should be remembered that joint destruction from urate deposition may be proceeding despite the fact that the patient has been made fairly comfortable. Prophylaxis should never be used in patients in whom the diagnosis has not been established. Even lower doses, such as 0.5 or 0.6 mg every other day, should be given to patients with renal insufficiency.

Pseudogout

Colchicine is used in pseudogout exactly as it is used in gout. If treated early, the acute attacks should respond to 2 mg intravenously just as well as would acute articular gout, but they will also respond to indomethacin and corticosteroids. Prevention of recurring attacks of pseudogout with colchicine is the only specific long-term therapy available for patients with CPPD deposition disease. In one preliminary study using doses similar to those used in gout, colchicine was very effective in preventing these attacks. The diagnosis of an attack of pseudogout is not necessarily an indication for prophylactic therapy, however. Many patients with CPPD deposition disease have such infrequent episodes of acute arthritis that it is difficult to justify taking a drug every day to prevent them; however, for patients disabled or inconvenienced by frequent attacks, the program is worth instituting.

Other Indications

Perhaps the most dramatically effective role for colchicine in the noncrystalline-induced arthropathies is in familial Mediterranean fever. Daily doses of 0.6 mg bid or tid have significantly reduced the number of recurring attacks (arthritis, fever, and serositis) in controlled studies. Amyloidosis is a common complication of familial Mediterranean fever and the most common cause of death in patients with it. It now appears that colchicine in the doses used for prophylaxis is predictably effective in preventing this complication; therefore, colchicine should be started with the first attack of the disease, even in children, and continued indefinitely. Dose adjustments will have to be made for children, in whom side effects may be more of a problem than in adults.

Preliminary uncontrolled observations have suggested that colchicine in doses of 0.6 mg bid or tid significantly enhances survival in patients with the more common forms of amyloidosis seen in this country. Particularly in AL or primary amyloidosis was duration of survival doubled compared to historical controls. No more effective therapy has been clearly documented; therefore, whatever else might be done, colchicine probably should be prescribed indefinitely for all patients with AL amyloidosis.

Colchicine may reduce the frequency of attacks in patients with Behçet's syndrome, but it does not seem to affect the outcome of the more serious ocular and CNS manifestations of the disease. In doses of about 1.2 mg/day, colchicine has been thought to benefit the skin in patients with systemic sclerosis, and it is widely used for that purpose. Although there are no adequate controlled studies, several open trials refute this claim. A recent small controlled study demonstrated the effectiveness of 0.5 mg of colchicine tid in patients with psoriatic arthritis, but the skin lesions did not benefit. Other rheumatic disease experiences are too preliminary to justify comment here, but this is a very versatile drug, and other indications for its use are likely to become apparent in the future.

CLINICAL ASPECTS OF SIDE EFFECTS AND CONTRAINDICATIONS

Major side effects of colchicine are listed in Table 5-2. In patients with normal hepatic and renal function and in oral doses less than 2 mg/day, the drug is usually very well tolerated, and no cumulative toxicity has been recognized. Occasional gastrointestinal complaints typically respond to temporary withdrawal or dose adjustments. Alopecia, sexual dysfunction, and stomatitis are rare. Major toxicity

Table 5-2. Side effects of colchicine

Common and usually not serious
   Gastrointestinal
      Nausea and vomiting
      Diarrhea
      Abdominal pain
   Local venous irritation (parenteral)

Less common and more serious
   Hemorrhagic gastroenteritis
   Aplastic anemia
   Disseminated intravascular coagulation
   CNS dysfunction
   Myopathy
   Hepatocellular failure
   Acute renal failure (with shock)
   Tissue necrosis (with extravasation)

Less common and less serious
   Alopecia
   Stomatitis
   Azoospermia
   Amenorrhea

most often results from standard doses given to patients with hepatic or renal insufficiency, or from excessive doses used to treat acute attacks of gout or pseudogout. Consequently severe toxicity is largely avoidable.

For daily therapy, as in the prophylaxis of acute articular gout, doses should be adjusted according to the degree of hepatic or renal dysfunction. Mild impairment might indicate no more than 0.6 mg once a day, and more severe impairment might indicate no more than 0.6 mg two or three times a week. Gastrointestinal side effects sometimes help determine dosages under these circumstances. Although routine laboratory toxicity monitoring is not widely employed in otherwise normal subjects, a monthly complete blood count might be prudent when the drug is given to patients with hepatic or renal insufficiency.

In the treatment of acute attacks of gout or pseudogout, it is best not to use colchicine at all when there is any significant hepatic or renal dysfunction. If the drug must be used in the face of mild renal insufficiency, 1-mg doses should be used intravenously with no more than 2 mg given in any 24-hour period. In terms of toxicity (and probably efficacy), parenteral colchicine should be considered to have at least twice the potency of the oral preparation. Hence the recommendation that no more than 4 mg be given intravenously in a 24-hour period. If an anti-inflammatory drug is required after the first 24 hours of intravenous colchicine therapy, some other agent, such as a NSAID, should be used.

Other contraindications to the use of colchicine include inflammatory bowel disease, pregnancy, and nursing mothers. It would be wise not to use therapeutic doses in patients with significant pre-existing gastrointestinal symptoms of any cause.

EXPENSE

Prophylactic oral colchicine is inexpensive. The 0.6-mg tablets will cost the patient about $0.15 each; the 0.5-mg tablets may be more expensive; therefore, gout or pseudogout prophylaxis should cost the patient no more than $0.30/day or about $9.00/month.

Antihyperuricemic Therapy

Above levels of 6.4–7.0 mg/dl, plasma is supersaturated with regard to uric acid, promoting urate deposition; below that level resorption of pre-existing urate deposits is promoted. Consequently the goal of antihyperuricemic therapy is to achieve a blood urate level less than 6.4 mg/dl, and to maintain it indefinitely. This goal can usually be accomplished with allopurinol, a drug that inhibits uric acid synthesis, and it can often be accomplished with any one of several agents that promote urate excretion. Currently two drugs are marketed in this country for the purpose of lowering serum uric acid by enhancing urate excretion: probenecid and sulfinpyrazone. A number of other available agents, including high-dose salicylates and diflunisal, share this uricosuric effect but are not generally used for that purpose.

INDICATIONS

Asymptomatic hyperuricemia is an elevated blood uric acid in a patient who has had no articular gout, clinically evident tophi, or documented urate-related kidney stones. In such a patient, the relatively low risk of developing gout, rarely a life-threatening disease and one that is treatable should it occur, hardly seems to justify the expense, inconvenience, and potential toxicity of an antihyperuricemic drug. Most informed opinion favors no therapy for asymptomatic hyperuricemia. Concerns are frequently expressed about the incidental finding of a very high blood uric acid level and its potential risk to the kidney, which, in fact, is rarely threatened except in the case of certain leukemias or the tumor lysis syndrome. If justified, these concerns may be addressed by calculating the uric acid–creatinine ratio from a spot urine sample; a ratio of less than 1 indicates no immediate threat of tubular precipitation and necrosis. In general the incidental finding of a very high blood uric acid in an asymptomatic patient requires more diagnostic than therapeutic attention.

Inhibition of urate synthesis by allopurinol is indicated in patients with certain tumors, particularly leukemias and lymphomas, before and during chemotherapy in order to prevent the acute renal damage that might result from the very high blood uric acid levels caused by the tumor lysis. The only other nongouty indication for antihyperuricemic therapy is in patients with hyperuricosuria (over 750–800 mg/24 hours) and recurrent calcium oxalate renal calculi; in this case urate might provide a nidus for stone formation. Obviously, allopurinol, and not a uricosuric agent, is used in this situation.

When to begin antihyperuricemic therapy and which drug to use in patients with documented gout are largely a matter of opinion. The long-term goal of such therapy is primarily to prevent tophaceous joint destruction, but recurring acute attacks of articular gout can be expected to cease, even without prophylactic colchicine, after the blood uric acid has been normalized for several months. Prevention of recurrent urate nephrolithiasis might also be a goal of therapy in some patients.

The first attack of articular gout usually announces the clinical onset of the disease. A second attack may not occur until years later even with no therapy, and it is unlikely that significant joint damage will accrue in the interval between the first and second attacks. Consequently many experienced clinicians will not treat the uric acid until after the second attack, but if this decision is made, prophylactic colchicine should not be prescribed after the first. Gout is sometimes first diagnosed in patients with severe and even terminal coexisting medical diseases. Since antihyperuricemic therapy is actually an investment in the future (prevention of joint destruction), patients with little or no future might not be considered appropriate candidates for such treatment. If the decision is made not to treat the uric acid in a gouty patient with a limited projected survival, prophylactic colchicine should be prescribed if frequent attacks have been a problem. Most rheumatologists would recommend antihyperuricemic therapy for all other patients with documented gout—after the second attack in those expected to live for several years.

A decision to treat the uric acid requires that a specific drug be chosen for this purpose, and the choice is primarily between allopurinol and a uricosuric agent. Although this choice is ultimately a matter of opinion in many cases, allopurinol is probably more toxic than the uricosuric drugs, but there may be specific reasons not to use them. Probenecid or sulfinpyrazone should not be prescribed in patients with a history of kidney stones unless it has been clearly documented that they are not urate related, and that is seldom the case. Patients with renal insufficiency will usually not respond to uricosuric drugs, and it might be wise not to try to enhance urate excretion in that case in any event. It is usually recommended that uricosuric agents not be given to the minority of gouty subjects who are already overexcreting uric acid (700–1000 mg/day on a normal purine diet). Finally it has been observed that patients with clinically evident tophi do not respond well to uricosuric agents, perhaps because of the large urate pool requiring mobilization, and allopurinol is usually recommended in that situation. Of course patients who fail to respond adequately to uricosuric drugs will require substitution of allopurinol. Since there is less apparent toxicity with probenecid or sulfinpyrazone, it would be reasonable to select one of these agents first in all other situations. Figure 5-4 summarizes an approach to antihyperuricemic therapy in patients with gout, and Table 5-3 compares the three antihyperuricemic agents available in this country. In no case should a drug affecting blood uric acid levels be given until the patient has completely recovered from an acute attack of articular gout. Lowering blood uric acid during an attack is very likely to worsen or prolong it.

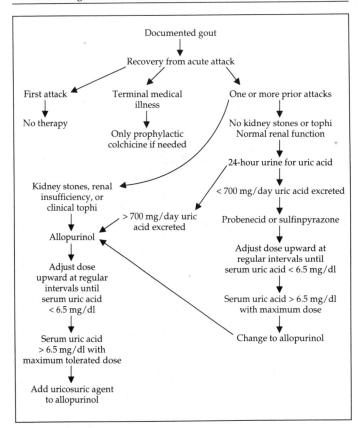

Fig. 5-4. Antihyperuricemic therapy in patients with gout.

Probenecid

Probenecid was discovered in the early 1950s as the consequence of an intentional search for agents that would interfere with the rapid renal excretion of penicillin. An almost incidental action was its effect on uric acid excretion, which turned out to be quite efficient, leading to its marketing as an antihyperuricemic agent.

Probenecid is available in 500-mg tablets as Benemid and it is available generically in the same tablet size. A combination of 500 mg of probenecid and 0.5 mg of colchicine is marketed as ColBENEMID, but fixed combinations such as this one are not recommended.

Table 5-3. Antihyperuricemic drugs available in the United States

Drug	Action	Dose schedule	Relative toxicity	Relative contraindications	Annual cost
Probenecid	Uricosuric	bid–tid	Low, mostly gastrointestinal	Renal insufficiency, nephrolithiasis, baseline uric acid overexcretion, tophaceous disease. Prior serious reaction.	Maximum dose: $288
Sulfinpyrazone	Uricosuric	bid–qid	Low, mostly gastrointestinal. Aplastic anemia may occur.	Renal insufficiency, nephrolithiasis, baseline uric acid overexcretion, tophaceous disease. (?) Peptic ulcer disease and prior serious reaction.	Maximum dose: $500
Allopurinol	Inhibits synthesis of uric acid	Once a day– bid (with larger doses)	Low-medium, severe "hypersensitivity" reaction uncommon	Prior serious reaction. Dose adjustments for renal insufficiency.	$91 for 300 mg/day; up to $275 for maximum dose

BASIC PHARMACOLOGY

General Properties and Mechanism

Probenecid is a lipid-soluble, weak, sulfur-containing organic acid (see Fig. 5-1) that can inhibit both the renal organic anion secretory transporter and the reabsorption transporter used by uric acid. Probenecid has **no** anti-inflammatory effects and therefore is unsuitable (alone) for acute gouty inflammation.

The renal secretory transporter is significantly more sensitive to inhibition than is the reabsorption transporter. Thus, low doses of the drug may inhibit only or predominantly secretion. Inhibition of secretion can result in elevation of blood urate levels. Two considerations are relevant to this observation. The first is that sufficiently high doses of probenecid must be used in order to inhibit the quantitatively more important reabsorption mechanism. The second is that even if doses sufficient to inhibit both transporters are used, drug concentration may be sufficiently low after initial doses, before plateau level is accomplished, that a transient effect on secretion only may occur. A transient increase in blood urate, possibly sufficient to cause precipitation, could result. This transient increase, and its potential for eliciting an acute gouty attack, provides one rationale for concomitant use of colchicine during early uricosuric therapy. Another rationale is increased mobilization of uric acid from sites of deposition as a result of the gradient created from these sites to blood as blood urate is decreased in response to uricosuria.

Mechanisms of Side Effects and Drug Interactions

Urate levels in tubular fluid increase as a result of probenecid therapy, in parallel with decreases in blood levels. Keeping in mind the previously indicated insolubility of uric acid and the effect of pH, at least the volume and theoretically the pH of urine should be kept elevated. The importance of this increases with increasing urate load (very high blood/tubular levels may be better handled with allopurinol; see Allopurinol).

Probenecid is well absorbed after oral administration and has a relatively short half-life. The latter represents combined influences of protein binding and renal secretion. As for any other weak organic acid, probenecid becomes increasingly ionized as pH increases; passive reabsorption of probenecid is limited and excretion favored by increased urinary pH (ion trapping). Thus, attempts to manipulate urinary pH to favor solubility of urate may simultaneously enhance excretion/decrease effect of probenecid.

Because many useful and commonly used drugs are also eliminated via the anion secretory transporter, significant potential exists for drug interactions; doses may have to be lowered to compensate for probenecid-induced increased blood concentrations of coadministered drugs. Blood levels of many members of the superfamily of sulfonamides are increased by probenecid, including thiazide diuretics (e.g., hydrochlorothiazide, chlorothiazide), oral hypoglycemic agents (glyburide, glypizide, chlorpropamide, tolbutamide), and sulfonamide antibiotics (e.g., sulfamethizole, sulfasalazine, and sulfisoxazole). NSAIDs are secreted via the transporter also, thus blood levels of NSAIDs may be significantly increased by probenecid coadministration (e.g., indomethacin, ketoprofen, meclofenamate acid). Since probenecid was designed to interfere with secretion of penicillins, it is fairly expected that levels as well as the half-lives of this class of antibiotics, and of the related cephalosporins, may be increased.

Weakly uricosuric NSAIDs (aspirin, diflunisal, salsalate and other salicylates, sulindac, possibly others) may antagonize the effectiveness of probenecid by competing with it. Antagonism by other drugs can likewise occur, e.g., pyrazinamide. Because probenecid is highly plasma protein bound ($\approx 90\%$), there is also potential for drug interactions via protein-binding displacement.

Toxicity is rare with probenecid. Hypersensitivity reactions may occur.

DOSING SCHEDULES

Once the patient has recovered from the acute attack of articular gout and has been taking prophylactic colchicine for a few days, probenecid is usually begun in a dose of 250 mg bid for a week, then increased to 500 mg bid. Even though it may not take that long for maximum effects to occur, it is usually suggested that the serum uric acid be remeasured two to four weeks after starting the 1 gm/day dose. If it is still greater than 6.5 mg/dl, the dose should be increased to 500 mg tid. After another few weeks, if the response is still inadequate, a total of 2000 mg/day is recommended, given in two or three divided doses. The manufacturers indicate that 2000 mg/day is the maximum dose, but some clinicians have prescribed as much as 3000 mg/day. If the blood uric acid has not responded adequately to 2000 mg/day, the drug probably should be abandoned in favor of allopurinol. If an adequate response has been obtained with 2000 mg/day or less, the serum uric acid should be rechecked every 6–12 months as the drug is continued indefinitely. Further dose adjustments are usually unnecessary, but sometimes it may be possible to reduce it after a year or longer of a normal serum uric acid.

Meanwhile uricosuric NSAIDs should be proscribed, since they interfere with the uricosuric effect of probenecid. An adequate fluid intake is especially important early in the course of therapy. Alkalization of the urine is often recommended with uricosuric drugs to increase urine urate solubility, but up to 7.5 gm/day of sodium bicarbonate or potassium citrate may be required to accomplish this, and potential benefits may not be worth the effort required. If there are concerns over the degree of uricosuria resulting from the therapy, a 24-hour urine uric acid determination might be reassuring.

CLINICAL ASPECTS OF SIDE EFFECTS, DRUG INTERACTIONS, AND CONTRAINDICATIONS

Probenecid does interfere with tubular transport and hence excretion of a number of pharmacologic agents; however, with the exception of the beta-lactams, this action is of doubtful clinical significance. Nonetheless, if an apparent reaction to one of these

Table 5-4. Reported probenecid side effects

Partially preventable
  Precipitation of acute articular gout
  Urate nephrolithiasis
Relatively common reactions
  Gastrointestinal symptoms
  Dermatitis
  Headache
  Drug fever
  Anaphylaxis
Rare reactions
  Hemolytic anemia
  Aplastic anemia
  Nephrotic syndrome
  Hepatic necrosis

agents occurs in a patient taking probenecid, appropriate dose adjustments should be made for the potentially offending drug.

Probenecid is generally well tolerated in doses of 2000 mg/day or less. Reported side effects are listed in Table 5-4. Precipitation of acute attacks of articular gout is partially preventable by the use of prophylactic colchicine, and urate nephrolithiasis is partially avoidable by appropriate patient selection and increased fluid intake and perhaps urine alkalization early in the course of therapy.

The most common side effects leading to drug withdrawal are gastrointestinal symptoms, which may occur sooner or later in up to 18% of patients taking the drug. Hypersensitivity reactions, including anaphylaxis, are much less common. The rare reactions are represented by only one, or a few, case reports. Several long-term experiences with probenecid have been reported, and toxicity withdrawal rates have ranged from 2–33%. A figure of 10% probably would be a fair average. No routine laboratory toxicity monitoring is required. No other absolute contraindications to probenecid exist except prior serious reactions to it; its safety in pregnancy is uncertain, however.

EXPENSE

Probenecid therapy is usually inexpensive. A 500-mg Benemid tablet will cost the patient about $0.40; the generic preparation costs about half that. Consequently, even with 2000 mg/day, the cost of a month's therapy can be as little as $24 and a year's as little as $288.

Sulfinpyrazone

Phenylbutazone is a potent NSAID with a weak uricosuric action. Because of its toxicity, various congeners were developed and evaluated during the 1950s in an effort to find a less toxic anti-inflammatory drug. These efforts lead to the discovery of sulfinpyrazone in the early 1960s. Although it is a potent uricosuric agent, sulfinpyrazone has no anti-inflammatory or analgesic effects, but it does share some of the toxicity of the parent compound. The drug is marketed only as a uricosuric agent for gout; it is available in 100-mg tablets and 200-mg capsules as Anturane, and it is available generically in the same forms.

BASIC PHARMACOLOGY

General Properties and Mechanism

Sulfinpyrazone is an analog of phenylbutazone (see chapter 2), a potent anti-inflammatory, effective uricosuric agent. (Sulfinpyrazone has some significant structural similarities to probenecid also, however; see Fig. 5-1). Sulfinpyrazone retains the uricosuric properties of its parent, but has no useful anti-inflammatory properties. The latter presents somewhat of a paradox in that platelet aggregation, which for many stimuli is dependent on arachidonic acid metabolism through cyclooxygenase, is very effectively inhibited by sulfinpyrazone. The difference could be due to different tissue sensitivities or other unknown mechanisms. One fortunate property of sulfinpyrazone is that it shares little of its parent's potentially serious effects on bone marrow; some gastrointestinal effects do occur, however.

The mechanism of uricosuric action of sulfinpyrazone is essentially identical to that of probenecid, although the intensity of effect is greater. Problems of potential biphasic dose effects, including initial low drug concentrations and decreased urate secretion, as well as considerations of urine pH and volume are likewise identical. The reader is thus referred to the initial section on excretion of uric acid and to the previous section on probenecid for details.

Mechanisms of Side Effects and Drug Interactions

Although the mechanism of effect is the same as probenecid, several similarities and some differences in other aspects are worthy of note. The effects of sulfinpyrazone on levels of other renally secreted drugs are very similar to the effects of probenecid; likewise, drugs that antagonize the uricosuric effects of probenecid also do so for sulfinpyrazone. Sulfinpyrazone is more extensively plasma protein bound than probenecid (c 99% versus 90%), and the potential for drug interactions via this route is greater. For example, increased free warfarin and warfarin effect can occur, further enhanced by sulfinpyrazone-elicited decreased metabolism of warfarin as well as by sulfinpyrazone's antiplatelet effects.

The duration of effect of sulfinpyrazone is significantly longer than that of probenecid. This is probably due to the small fraction of sulfinpyrazone that is converted to an active metabolite, thus increasing intensity and duration of effect. Sulfinpyrazone is mostly ionized at all usually encountered pH values in the body; its excretion is thus not enhanced by changes in urinary pH.

DOSING SCHEDULES

After the patient has recovered from the acute episode of articular gout, and after several days of prophylactic colchicine, sulfinpyrazone is usually started in doses of 100 mg bid and then increased to 200 mg bid a week later. Thereafter the dose is increased by 100-mg increments every one to four weeks (depending on patient and physician convenience) until the serum uric acid is less than 6.5 mg/dl or until a total dose of 800 mg/day is achieved. Above 400 mg/day, the drug should be given in three or four equally divided doses. If 800 mg/day is inadequate, the drug should be abandoned in favor of allopurinol. Once a satisfactory response is achieved, that dose is continued indefinitely with blood uric acid measurements every 6–12 months. Occasionally it is possible to reduce the dose late in the course of therapy.

As with probenecid, uricosuric NSAIDs are avoided and the patient should be well hydrated, especially early in the course of therapy. Urine alkalization might be considered under certain circumstances but is difficult to accomplish and may not be worth the effort.

CLINICAL ASPECTS OF SIDE EFFECTS, DRUG INTERACTIONS, AND CONTRAINDICATIONS

Sulfinpyrazone has not been as well investigated as probenecid in terms of its effect on the renal tubular transport of other drugs. For reasons that may be related to other actions, the drug has been reported to potentiate the action of sulfonamides, sulfonylurias, insulin, and warfarin. It can be expected to precipitate acute gouty arthritis and urate-related nephrolithiasis with the same frequency as probenecid, and the same precautions are indicated.

The most common side effects are gastrointestinal symptoms that are about as frequent as with probenecid. There is concern that sulfinpyrazone may cause, reactivate, or interfere with the healing of peptic ulcer disease, and active or pre-existing ulcer disease is considered a contraindication. It is not yet clear whether or not the drug may actually induce a gastropathy similar to that caused by the NSAIDs. Other serious side effects related to its ability to inhibit prostaglandin synthesis have not yet been observed. Rashes are uncommon, and blood dyscrasias have been reported less often than might be expected, considering the parent compound, phenylbutazone; however, bone marrow aplasia has occurred and periodic complete blood counts are recommended as long as the therapy is continued. Despite these concerns, sulfinpyrazone is widely regarded as better tolerated than probenecid. In addition to peptic ulcer disease, the drug is contraindicated in patients with previous serious reactions to it or to phenylbutazone and in patients with blood dyscrasias. Its safety in pregnancy is not established.

A potentially beneficial side effect is under investigation. Presumably because of the ability of sulfinpyrazone to inhibit platelet prostaglandin synthesis, it exerts an antiplatelet effect in vitro and in vivo. Clinical applications of this action are being explored.

EXPENSE

Sulfinpyrazone can be expected to be somewhat more expensive than probenecid. Anturane costs the patient about $0.40 for a 100-mg tablet and $0.60 for a 200-mg capsule; the generic preparations cost about half that. Assuming four complete blood counts a year for toxicity monitoring, a final dose of 800 mg/day and the use of the generic preparation, a year's therapy will cost the patient about $500 ($440 for the drug and $60 for the laboratory monitoring).

Allopurinol

Allopurinol is an analog of hypoxanthine. It was synthesized in the 1960s with antineoplastic effects in mind (it prolongs the action of 6-mercaptopurine [6MP]). Although it demonstrated no antitumor activity, it was found in the laboratory to be an inhibitor of xanthine oxidase and in human subjects to be an effective antihyperuricemic agent, the action for which it was ultimately marketed. Allopurinol continues to be the only drug available in this country that efficiently lowers blood uric acid through a nonrenal mechanism. It is sold in 100-mg and 300-mg tablets as Zyloprim and is available generically in tablets of the same size.

BASIC PHARMACOLOGY

General Properties and Mechanism

As indicated in the main introduction to this section, allopurinol was developed to interfere with the metabolism of 6MP and thus prolong its duration in vivo. As can be seen in Fig. 5-5, allopurinol is a structural analog of naturally occurring purine metabolites that are substrates for the enzyme xanthine oxidase, which also converts 6MP to an inactive metabolite. Allopurinol competitively inhibits the enzyme and also interacts with it much as its usual substrates. Indeed, allopurinol can be converted to an active metabolite, oxypurinol (oxipurinol; alloxanthine) by the enzyme (Fig. 5-5).

Allopurinol is classified as a "suicide substrate," i.e., a substrate converted by the enzyme to a reactive species that then inactivates the enzyme. The half-life of oxypurinol is longer than the half-life of allopurinol. The latter is in part due to reabsorption of oxypurinol by the same renal transporter used by urate. Oxypurinol could thus competitively antagonize urate reabsorption as well, although this is not usually indicated to be part of allopurinol's total antihyperuricemic mechanism. Neither allopurinol nor oxypurinol is renally secreted.

Of the several consequences of the inhibition of xanthine oxidase by allopurinol/oxypurinol, the most important is directly decreased production of uric acid. As pointed out in the initial section on uric acid production, both xanthine and hypoxanthine, unlike uric acid, can be salvaged and reused in nucleic acid synthesis, thus effectively removing them. Products of xanthine/hypoxanthine salvage (IMP, AMP, GMP) decrease de novo purine synthesis through feedback inhibition of synthetic enzymes. Additional decreases in de novo synthesis may result through the formation of 5'-allopurinol ribonucleotide, with depletion of a necessary precursor (5'-phosphoribosylpyrophosphate). Thus, allopurinol can indirectly reduce purines available for conversion to uric acid.

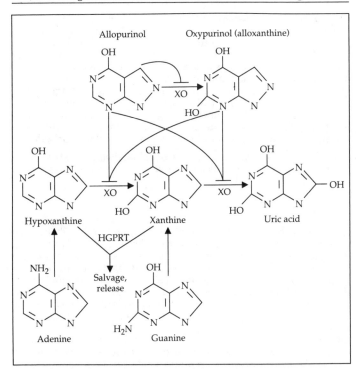

Fig. 5-5. Pathways of purine metabolism in humans. Allopurinol and its active metabolite inhibit xanthine oxidase (XO), resulting in decreased uric acid via redistribution to xanthine and hypoxanthine. The latter have independent solubilities and are also utilized in the purine salvage pathways. Allopurinol inhibits its own metabolism, which can actually shorten effect duration (see text). (—, inhibits; HGPRT, hypoxanthine-guanine phosphoribosyl transferase.)

Though both xanthine and hypoxanthine, like uric acid, are relatively insoluble, these compounds exhibit independent solubilities. This means that the total quantity of purines that can be solubilized can be increased by distribution among the forms rather than to a single form only.

Allopurinol can be used to circumvent hyperuricemia in circumstances of large-scale cell lysis such as might occur as a result of radiation or chemotherapy. Use in this context prevents excess levels of urate in the renal tubules as well as in blood, simultaneously minimizing the possibility of an acute inflammatory episode and the possibility of intratubular precipitation and loss of renal function.

Mechanisms of Side Effects and Drug Interactions

Allopurinol is rapidly and effectively absorbed after oral administration. Allopurinol does not bind to plasma proteins to any significant extent, thus drug interactions via this route are unlikely.

Allopurinol does interfere with the metabolism of 6MP, in accordance with the purpose for which it was designed. It should be remembered that azathioprine is inactive and is converted in vivo to 6MP. Thus, the effects of both 6MP and azathioprine can be intensified and prolonged if administered simultaneously with allopurinol, and dose adjustments may be necessary. Allopurinol may inhibit hepatic drug biotransformation, which may be of significance for some drugs. Coadministration of allopurinol and probenecid may necessitate adjustments in the dosages of both (up, down, respectively); without adjustment, probenecid may interfere with reabsorption of oxypurinol, thus decreasing overall allopurinol effect.

The direct side effects of allopurinol include abdominal distress, liver dysfunction, and skin rashes (hypersensitivity?). The mechanisms are not well described.

DOSING SCHEDULE

Because of the long half-life of allopurinol, and its metabolite oxypurinol, the drug can be given once a day but twice-daily dosage schedules have been recommended for patients requiring more than 300 mg/day. The usual initial dose is 300 mg/day begun after recovery from acute articular gout and after a few days of prophylactic colchicine. Lower doses should be used in patients with renal insufficiency. If renal function is mildly to moderately impaired, the beginning dose is 200 to 100 mg/day; for severely impaired renal function, 100 mg should be given every two to three days. After about a week of the initial dose, serum uric acid is remeasured and appropriate upward dose adjustments made if the value is greater than 6.5 mg/dl. Further dose adjustments can be made weekly or at the convenience of the patient and the physician. For patients with normal renal function, the usual dose increments are 100 mg each. In most cases, 300 mg/day will be adequate, and 800 mg/day is the maximum dose recommended by the manufacturers; however, doses larger than 800 mg/day are sometimes required in cases of severe tophaceous gout and might be prescribed with caution. Alternatively a uricosuric agent might be added to the program if large doses of allopurinol are necessary and there is no nephrolithiasis. Allopurinol will prolong the half-life of probenecid, and 1000 mg/day of this agent might be adequate to normalize the blood uric acid in patients who have incompletely responded to 600 mg/day or more of allopurinol. In cases of severe tophaceous gout, it might be desirable to lower the blood uric acid to less than 3 mg/dl. This will hasten urate mobilization and resorption of tophi. This goal can be recommended whenever it can be achieved with 600 mg/day or less of the drug.

It is generally understood that an adequate dose of allopurinol, once it is achieved, is continued indefinitely. After the daily requirement is established, blood uric acid levels should be checked about every six months to be certain that adequate control is maintained. After clinically evident tophi have disappeared, a lower dose might be possible and could be attempted. A year or longer is usually required for resolution of tophi. The question of stopping antihyperuricemic therapy years after tophaceous resolution has been raised, but this practice is not recommended now, though it might be acceptable in the very elderly and those with terminal illnesses.

CLINICAL ASPECTS OF SIDE EFFECTS, DRUG INTERACTIONS, AND CONTRAINDICATIONS

Allopurinol will interfere with the metabolism of azathioprine, 6MP, and other purine analogs, and these agents should be given in much smaller doses and with great caution to patients taking allopurinol. For reasons that are not clear, the toxicity of other cytotoxic agents, such as cyclophosphamide, is also enhanced by allopurinol; so any cytotoxic agent should be used with caution in patients taking it. Because of an inhibitory effect on hepatic microsomal enzymes, allopurinol may delay the metabolism of dicumarol, sulfonylureas, and probenecid. An increased incidence of skin rashes due to ampicillin and amoxicillin has been reported in patients taking allopurinol. Severe reactions to the drug may occur more frequently in patients also taking thiazide diuretics.

Xanthine renal stones and oxypurinol crystal deposition disease might be expected in patients taking allopurinol but rarely have been reported. Of course acute attacks of articular gout do occur commonly early in the course of therapy, especially in patients not taking prophylactic colchicine. If an attack does occur, the allopurinol should not be discontinued; the resulting rise in serum uric acid will further aggravate the situation.

Allopurinol toxicity is summarized in Table 5-5. The drug is usually well tolerated with a toxicity withdrawal rate as low as 5%; however, some type of reaction is reported by about 20% of patients taking the drug, though the reported reaction is often no more than an acute attack of gouty arthritis. Toxicity is enhanced by renal insufficiency (often related to excessive doses) and concomitant use of ampicillin, amoxicillin, and thiazide diuretics. Gastrointestinal symptoms may be minimized by taking the drug with food; they should rarely lead to its withdrawal. Skin reactions are most often widespread pruritic maculopapular rashes and diffuse pruritic swelling of the hands, feet, and sometimes face. Although it is not always necessary to stop the drug when these rashes occur, they may herald a more severe reaction, and it is probably prudent to at least temporarily interrupt therapy. Antihistamines are often effective treatment. Likewise abnormal liver tests may be trivial but may also be the first sign of a serious reaction, especially if there is a cholestatic picture.

The most dreaded reaction to the drug has been called the "allopurinol hypersensitivity reaction," a clinical syndrome usually consisting of a severe dermatitis (typically toxic epidermal necrolysis), fever, renal failure or worsening renal function, and varying degrees of hepatitis, eosinophilia, and leukocytosis. Histologically a vasculitis may occur. Not all components are always present, and a broad spectrum of severity has been reported, but the overall mortality rate has been about 20%. Risk factors for the reaction include preexisting renal insufficiency (often with excessive doses of allopurinol prescribed) and concomitant use of thiazide diuretics. It most often appears in the first few weeks of therapy. Any suggestion that this

Table 5-5. Allopurinol side effects

Common and usually not serious
  Precipitation of acute articular gout
  Rashes
  Nausea
  Diarrhea
  Abnormal liver tests
Uncommon and potentially serious
  Toxic epidermal necrolysis with or without the "allopurinol
    hypersensitivity reaction"
  Bone marrow suppression
  Hepatitis
  Sarcoid-like reaction
  Vasculitis
  Peripheral neuropathy
  Renal failure
  Oxypurinol crystal deposition
  Xanthine nephrolithiasis
  Cataracts

syndrome may be developing should lead to immediate drug withdrawal. High-dose corticosteroid therapy has been reported to be beneficial.

Bone marrow depression, isolated hepatitis, a sarcoid-like reaction, a more limited vasculitis, peripheral neuropathy, and isolated renal failure apparently due to allopurinol have been reported rarely. The isolated renal failure has usually been in the context of tumor lysis.

The only laboratory toxicity monitoring recommended routinely is periodic liver tests in patients with prior liver disease and periodic tests of renal function to be certain that dose reductions are not indicated. A fever or rash developing during the course of therapy should lead to a complete blood count and hepatic and renal function tests.

The only absolute contraindication to allopurinol is a prior serious reaction to it, usually in the form of the "hypersensitivity" syndrome. There are too few experiences with the drug in women of child-bearing age to know whether or not it is safe to use during pregnancy and in nursing mothers. Animal studies have been reassuring, however.

EXPENSE

Allopurinol therapy can be quite inexpensive. Zyloprim costs the patient about $0.25 for the 100-mg tablet and about $0.50 for the 300-mg size. Generic allopurinol costs about half that; therefore, considering no toxicity monitoring is necessary, a year of therapy at 300 mg/day can cost as little as $91, not counting the laboratory tests that go into establishing the correct dose. Considering the potential devastation that can result from severe tophaceous gout, this may be one of the most cost-effective therapies in all of medicine.

Bibliography

OVERVIEWS

Diamond, H. S. Control of crystal-induced arthropathies. *Rheum. Dis. Clin. North Am.* 15:557–567, 1989.

Kelley, W. N. Antihyperuricemic Drugs. In W. N. Kelley et al. (eds.), *Textbook of Rheumatology* (3rd ed.). Philadelphia: Saunders, 1989, Pp. 889–904.

Wortmann, R. L. Management of Hyperuricemia. In D. J. McCarty (ed.), *Arthritis and Allied Conditions. A Textbook of Rheumatology* (11th ed.). Philadelphia: Lea & Febiger, 1989. Pp. 1677–1690.

COLCHICINE

Ahern, M. J., et al. Does colchicine work? The results of the first controlled study in acute gout. *Aust. N.Z. J. Med.* 17:301–304, 1987.

Famaey, J. P. Colchicine in therapy. State of the art and new perspectives for an old drug. *Clin. Exp. Rheumatol.* 6:305–317, 1988.

Gupta, R. S., and Dudani, A. K. Mechanism of action of antimitotic drugs: A new hypothesis based on the role of cellular calcium. *Med. Hypotheses* 28:57–69, 1989.

Spilberg, I., et al. Mechanism of action of colchicine in acute urate crystal-induced arthritis. *J. Clin. Invest.* 64:775–780, 1979.

Wallace, S. L., and Singer, J. Z. Review: Systemic toxicity associated with the intravenous administration of colchicine—guidelines for use. *J. Rheumatol.* 15:495–499, 1988.

Wallace, S. L., et al. Renal function predicts colchicine toxicity: guidelines for the prophylactic use of colchicine in gout. *J. Rheumatol.* 18:264–269, 1991.

Yu, T. The efficacy of colchicine prophylaxis in articular gout—a reappraisal after 20 years. *Semin. Arthritis Rheum.* 12:256–264, 1982.

URICOSURIC AGENTS

Ali, M., and McDonald, W. D. Effects of sulfinpyrazone on platelet prostaglandin synthesis and platelet release of serotonin. *J. Lab. Clin. Med.* 89:868, 1977.

Boger, W. P., and Strickland, S. C. Probenecid (Benemid). Its use and side-effects in 2502 patients. *Arch. Intern. Med.* 95:83, 1955.

Kippen, I., Whitehouse, M. W., and Klinenberg, J. R. Pharmacology of uricosuric drugs. *Ann. Rheum. Dis.* 33:391, 1974.

Rosenkranz, B., et al. Effects of sulfinpyrazone on renal function and prostaglandin formation in man. *Nephron* 39:237–243, 1985.

Thompson, C. R., et al. Long-term uricosuric therapy in gout. *Arthritis Rheum.* 5:384, 1962.

ALLOPURINOL

Boston Collaborative Drug Surveillance Program. Excess of ampicillin rashes associated with allopurinol or hyperuricemia. *N. Engl. J. Med.* 286:505–507, 1972.

Bull, P. W., and Scott, J. T. Intermittent control of hyperuricemia in the treatment of gout. *J. Rheumatol.* 16:1246–1248, 1989.

Edwards, N. L., et al. Enhanced purine salvage during allopurinol therapy: an important pharmacologic property in humans. *J. Lab. Clin. Med.* 98:673, 1981.

Elion, G. Nobel lecture in physiology of medicine—1988: The purine path to chemotherapy. *In Vitro Cell. Dev. Biol.* 25:321–330, 1989.

Ettinger, B., et al. Randomized trial of allopurinol in the prevention of calcium oxalate calculi. *N. Engl. J. Med.* 315:1386–1389, 1986.

Hande, K. R., Noone, R. M., and Stone, W. J. Severe allopurinol toxicity. *Am. J. Med.* 76:47–56, 1984.

McInnes, G. T., Lawson, D. H., and Jick, H. Acute adverse reactions atributed to allopurinol in hospitalised patients. *Ann. Rheum. Dis.* 40:245–249, 1981.

Singer, J. Z., and Wallace, S. L. The allopurinol hypersensitivity syndrome. *Arthritis Rheum.* 29:82–87, 1986.

6

Drug Therapy of Specific Rheumatic Diseases

This chapter contains a brief overview of the drug therapy of individual rheumatic diseases, with the emphasis on the more common ones. Most of the drugs mentioned in this chapter have been discussed elsewhere in this book, but a few have not been specifically addressed; these include the simple analgesics, the antidepressant drugs, and various agents with a vasodilating action. Overall these drugs are more widely used in fields other than rheumatology, and they have been discussed in detail in other handbooks in this series. When appropriate, dosage schedules and side effects briefly will be detailed. The classification of rheumatic diseases outlined in Table 1-1 (p. 2) will be followed.

Connective Tissue Diseases

RHEUMATOID ARTHRITIS

The drug therapy of rheumatoid arthritis (RA) is determined by the degree of disease activity and the apparent disease severity (or prognosis). Indicators of disease activity and severity are listed in Table 6-1. RA displays a broad spectrum of severity, and the disease activity typically waxes and wanes over varying periods of time. Consequently careful initial and periodic follow-up assessments are crucial in designing appropriate drug programs. In most patients the pattern of disease severity is established after the first year or so, but activity can still fluctuate, even in patients with severe disease.

General Approaches to Therapy

The generally available therapeutic approaches to the patient with RA are outlined in Table 6-2. This table emphasizes that drug therapy is only one aspect of overall disease management, and sometimes it is not the most important one. Traditionally the management of RA is illustrated by a pyramid model; an example is provided in Fig. 6-1. However, this model has a number of defects and its value is currently debated. Perhaps the major defect in this and other pyramid models is that the behavior of the disease often precludes following the logical stepwise progression that they imply. Not all patients who need methotrexate will need surgery or systemic corticosteroids or even joint injections, and corticosteroids should not be considered definitive therapy (on a par with auranofin) in any event. The defects in the pyramid model need not detract from the fact that the drug therapy of RA is usually stepwise and

Table 6-1. Assessment of disease activity and severity (or prognosis) in patients with RA

Indicators of disease activity
  Joint pain (especially at rest)
  Degree and duration of morning stiffness
  Weight loss
  Number and magnitude of swollen and tender joints on physical exam[a]
  Joint function as measured by grip strength and walking time
  Elevated acute-phase reactants (or increased erythrocyte sedimentation rate)
  Anemia of chronic disease
  Progression of erosive changes on joint radiographs
  Extra-articular features except Sjögren's syndrome and subcutaneous nodules
Indicators of severe disease (or a poor prognosis)
  Widespread active arthritis (more than 10–12 simultaneously swollen and tender joints)[b]
  Subcutaneous nodules[b]
  Strongly positive test for rheumatoid factor[b]
  Early appearance and rapid progression of erosive changes on joint radiographs[b]
  Other serologic abnormalities such as antinuclear antibodies or circulating immune complexes[b]
  Limited formal education[b]
  Eosinophilia[b]
  Joint deformity
  Significant functional impairment
  Other extra-articular features than Sjögren's syndrome
  Disease-related death

[a]Probably the most reliable single indicator of active disease.
[b]Often apparent early in the course of the disease and useful as prognostic indicators.

Table 6-2. General therapeutic approaches to the patient with RA

Verbal
  Education
  Reassurance
  Support
Physical
  Relief of symptoms
  Education
  Prevention of disability
  Reversal of disability
  Correction of deformities
  Orthotics
Drugs
  Simple analgesics
  Anti-inflammatory agents
  Slow-acting agents
Surgical
  Prophylactic (synovectomy)
  Reconstructive (including joint replacement)

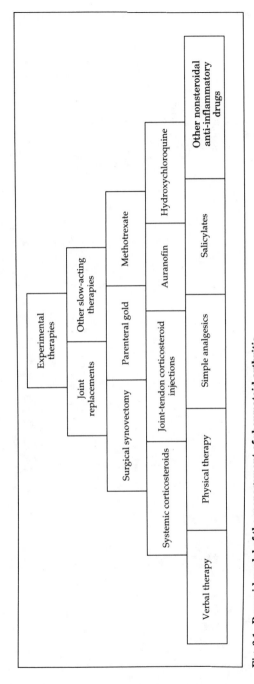

Fig. 6-1. Pyramid model of the management of rheumatoid arthritis.

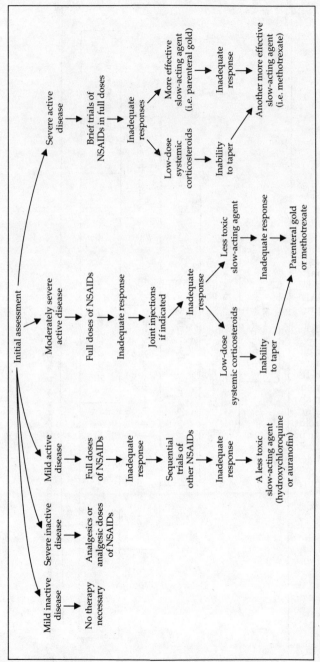

Fig. 6-2. Progression of drug therapy in patients with rheumatoid arthritis.

progressive; however, the progression is just difficult to diagram, but an attempt is made in Fig. 6-2.

Nonsteroidal Anti-inflammatory Drugs

Unless contraindicated, the usual first step in the drug management of symptomatic RA is a nonsteroidal anti-inflammatory drug (NSAID). For patients with no or minimally active disease, analgesic doses might be recommended, but when significant disease activity exists, a satisfactory response will usually require anti-inflammatory doses—often maximum anti-inflammatory doses. Because of their several advantages, salicylates would be a reasonable first choice, with other NSAIDs tried sequentially if salicylates are not tolerated or fail to be adequately beneficial. Because of its side effects and lack of specific advantages in RA, indomethacin should not be an initial or early choice. Two weeks of a maximum dose of any NSAID is probably an adequate trial. Even if a satisfactory response is never achieved with any NSAID, one that is well tolerated should probably be continued as long as active disease is present. Although disease outcome may not be affected, this practice should result in lowering the required doses of analgesics and systemic corticosteroids. Once a complete remission in disease activity has occurred spontaneously or secondary to slow-acting drug therapy, the NSAID can be withdrawn gradually. If the disease activity returns, the NSAID can be restarted immediately with no permanent harm having resulted from its withdrawal.

Corticosteroids

For patients with moderately to severely active disease despite adequate trials of NSAIDs and for patients with active disease in whom NSAIDs are contraindicated, low-dose systemic corticosteroid therapy should be started. If not already underway, serious consideration should be given to beginning slow-acting drug therapy to allow for corticosteroid withdrawal in the near future. Systemic corticosteroids should not be regarded as definitive long-term therapy; their purpose is to tide the patient over until time or another drug leads to lessened disease activity. Unless NSAIDs are contraindicated, corticosteroids are added on to an ongoing NSAID program. In rheumatology practices, about one-third of patients with RA will require courses of corticosteroids.

Slow-Acting Agents

Seldom does any true urgency exist in reaching a decision to begin slow-acting drug (SAARD) therapy, though it is often apparent at the time of the patient's first visit that one of these agents will be indicated. The decision is based largely on disease severity or prognosis and disease activity in the face of adequate anti-inflammatory drug therapy; however, a legitimate need for systemic corticosteroids implies disease activity even if none is clinically apparent. The more equivocal the indications for SAARD therapy, the longer the decision can be delayed, and, once made, in this case one of the least toxic drugs should be used first. Current opinion, however, seems to favor more aggressive **early** therapy in an attempt to prevent the irreversible joint damage that tends to begin in the first year or two of the disease in what may be the majority of patients. After the SAARD is started, ongoing NSAID or corticosteroid therapy, or both, is continued as long as active disease is present. A satisfactory SAARD is continued indefinitely or as long as it is tolerated. Withdrawal can lead to a disease flare that may prove more difficult to manage than the original process.

Analgesics

Patients with active RA most often require (or request) analgesics to use on an as-needed basis, and these agents may be the only drugs indicated with inactive disease and previously damaged joints that lead to mechanical pain. NSAIDs are probably the most effective analgesics in RA, but they may be neither effective nor safe in patients already taking maximum doses of another NSAID, and that is the usual situation. Consequently no really satisfactory analgesic can be recommended for most patients.

Perhaps the best choice is acetaminophen, but concern lingers over the possibility of an analgesic abuse pattern of nephritis in subjects who regularly consume combinations of NSAIDs and acetaminophen; however, few reported observations have documented this occurrence. For occasional use with NSAIDs, up to 2 gm/day of acetaminophen is probably safe. Codeine in a dose of 30–60 mg is also effective, but side effects are frequent and the drug is habit-forming. Codeine analogs such as dihydrocodeine and oxycodone are probably equally effective but have the same disadvantages. Propoxyphene and its various analogs are less effective analgesics, but they generally have fewer side effects. In practice combinations of acetaminophen with propoxyphene analogs (Darvocet-N) and codeine analogs (Tylox, Tylenol with codeine) are widely prescribed but have not been adequately studied in the context of RA with or without simultaneous NSAID therapy. If these agents are to be prescribed, strict limitations should be placed on their use and every possible precaution employed to guard against drug abuse. Patients should clearly understand that the analgesic is for occasional use and is not a mainstay of the therapeutic program. The more potent narcotics should never be used in the routine management of RA.

Tentative evidence suggests that some antidepressant drugs, primarily amitriptyline, may have a beneficial effect on many of the rheumatic symptoms experienced by patients with RA. Amitriptyline doses have usually been in the range of only 25–50 mg, most often given only at night. Side effects from these low doses are usually minimal; nightmares, dry mouth, and morning drowsiness have been the major problems. Especially for patients who report disturbed sleep due to symptoms of the disease, a low-dose nocturnal antidepressant might be indicated. These agents are probably more effective than hypnotic-sedative drugs and are not habit-forming. Alternatively cyclobenzaprine might be tried for patients intolerant of antidepressants, but no studies have addressed its effectiveness in RA.

Extra-articular Manifestations

Serious extra-articular manifestations of RA may require more aggressive therapy than does the active joint disease. Probably the most serious of these is an arteritis resembling polyarteritis nodosa. Some experiences have suggested that it may respond to D-penicillamine given in varying dosage schedules, but combinations of oral or bolus intravenous cyclophosphamide and high-dose corticosteroids appear to be more effective. No generally accepted standard dosage schedule exists for either the cyclophosphamide or the corticosteroids. Amyloidosis secondary to RA is another life-threatening extra-articular manifestation, and it may partially respond to oral colchicine or cytotoxic immunosuppressive drugs, but there are few published experiences. The drug therapy of Felty's syndrome is controversial; high-dose corticosteroids and lithium may increase the peripheral neutrophil count, but they do not seem to favorably influence the infection rate. Rheumatoid pericarditis and pleuritis are seldom life threatening and both may respond to indomethacin. If indomethacin fails or is not tolerated, about 30 mg/day of prednisone is usually effective. No drug therapy has proven beneficial for rheumatoid lung disease, though short courses of high-dose corticosteroids are often tried empirically when the process appears to be rapidly progressive. Anecdotal reports have indicated improvement with slow-acting drug therapy, particularly parenteral gold and D-penicillamine.

SYSTEMIC LUPUS ERYTHEMATOSUS

Many, if not most, of the drug therapies used by rheumatologists in patients with systemic lupus erythematosus (SLE) are empiric. Although considerable medical literature addresses the subject, little of it is really scientific. A number of problems exist in designing and carrying out scientific drug studies in patients with SLE. Disease expressions and their severity vary widely from patient to patient, making it difficult to study the effects of any drug in a homogeneous population. Furthermore, disease activity in any one patient may fluctuate markedly over varying periods of time, making it difficult to distinguish a drug action from the natural course of the disease. It is frequently not even certain that an apparent flare in disease activity is due to SLE; infections occur often in these patients and they are often confused with active disease. Finally systemic corticosteroids have become so firmly entrenched as a mainstay of therapy that controlled studies of their efficacy are widely regarded as unethical.

General Principles of Therapy

There are a few generally accepted principles to follow in managing patients with SLE. No routine drug therapy exists for the disease itself; usually the specific individual manifestations are treated. Aggressive therapy is reserved for serious disease expressions; manifestations that do not threaten organs or life are treated symptomatically. Inactive disease may require no therapy; however, drugs should be withdrawn very carefully in patients who appear to have recovered from a serious manifestation. Two or more manifestations often flare together, and therapy is determined by the most serious of them. The drugs most often used for serious expressions of the disease have potentially serious side effects, and this should temper therapeutic enthusiasm. Infection is the most common cause of death in patients with SLE, and the infection rate may be related more to the drug therapy of the disease than to the disease itself. Although the survival rates in patients with SLE have improved remarkably over the past 50 years, it is uncertain that the drug therapy of the disease has been the cause. In fact, good general medical care may be as important to disease outcome as are the various drugs used for specific manifestations of it. Early detection and appropriate therapy of infections are especially important.

Four groups of drugs are widely used for the treatment of SLE manifestations: NSAIDs, antimalarials, corticosteroids, and immunosuppressive agents including azathioprine and cyclophosphamide. In no case is the role for any one or combination of these agents absolutely defined; their indications remain a matter of opinion. The following discussion will attempt to present a relatively balanced version of patterns of therapy prevalent in 1991. Some approaches to common individual disease manifestations are summarized in Table 6-3. Each group of agents will be discussed briefly from the viewpoint of its use in SLE.

NSAIDs

Since nephritis is prevalent in patients with SLE, NSAIDs are often contraindicated. If NSAIDs must be used in patients with nephritis, low doses of a nonacetylated salicylate would be a wise choice. These agents are most useful in managing arthralgias, arthritis, and low-grade fever due to the disease. They are also frequently beneficial in the treatment of symptomatic pleuritis or pericarditis; indomethacin tends to be a superior drug in these situations if there are no contraindications to its use. A NSAID will seldom be required indefinitely, and periodic attempts to withdraw it should be made.

Antimalarials

It is widely believed that antimalarials exert some beneficial effects on the relatively minor extracutaneous manifestations of SLE, such as arthralgias, low-grade fever, and constitutional symptoms; studies attempting to document these benefits are underway; however, the most obvious role for the antimalarials in SLE is in the context of serious cutaneous involvement, especially discoid and subacute cutaneous lupus. There is also convincing recent evidence that maintenance hydroxychloroquine (HCQ) can actually prevent disease flares, suggesting that there may be a role for its sustained use in patients who have frequent exacerbations affecting any organ system. HCQ is used almost exclusively in this country and generally in doses similar to those used in RA. An initial dose of 400–600 mg/day is followed by a maintenance dose of 200–400 mg/day as soon as a clinical response becomes apparent. The response is often apparent earlier in cutaneous lupus than it is in RA. Side effects and precautions are the same in SLE as in RA.

Systemic Corticosteroids

Systemic corticosteroids continue to be the mainstay of the drug therapy of SLE, especially in the context of its more serious manifestations. When used to treat relatively minor symptomatic manifestations, the lowest possible dose should be used, but frequent

Table 6-3. Systemic drug therapy of common individual manifestations of systemic lupus erythematosus

Manifestation	Initial management	Short-term management	Long-term management
Nonspecific constitutional symptoms	None **OR** prednisone 10 mg/day or less	Taper prednisone by 1 mg every 1–2 weeks to none or to lowest dose required to control symptoms	None **OR** taper prednisone to every other day if required and successful **OR** hydroxychloroquine
Fever (exclude infection)	NSAIDs **OR** prednisone 10–15 mg/day, gradually increasing to whatever dose required to suppress fever; dose q8–12h often necessary initially	Depends on dose; taper rapidly to 15 mg/day, then by 1.0–2.5 mg every 1–2 weeks to none or to every other day if necessary and successful	Usually none required **OR** NSAIDs **OR** every-other-day prednisone if successful **OR** hydroxychloroquine
Arthritis/arthralgia	NSAIDs **OR** prednisone 15 mg/day or less; doses q8–12h often necessary	Taper prednisone by 1.0–2.5 mg every 1–2 weeks to none or to every other day if necessary and successful	Usually none required **OR** NSAIDs **OR** every-other-day prednisone if successful **OR** hydroxychloroquine
Cutaneous including discoid and subacute cutaneous lupus (photosensitivity and malar rashes may require no systemic therapy)	Hydroxychloroquine 400–600 mg/day **AND/OR** prednisone 15 mg/day or less	When stable attempt to reduce hydroxychloroquine to 200 mg/day; taper prednisone by 1.0–2.5 mg every 1–2 weeks to none or to every other day if successful and necessary	Maintain hydroxychloroquine 200–400 mg/day until several months after clearing of active lesions or indefinitely
Serositis (pleuritis or pericarditis or both)	Indomethacin 150 mg/day **OR** prednisone 15–30 mg/day as necessary	Trial of indomethacin withdrawal when asymptomatic **OR** taper prednisone depending on dose —rapidly to 15 mg/day, then by 1.0–2.5 mg every 1–2 weeks to none or to every other day if necessary and successful	Usually none required **OR** indomethacin **OR** every-other-day prednisone if necessary and successful

Table 6-3. Systemic drug therapy of common individual manifestations of systemic lupus erythematosus (continued)

Manifestation	Initial management	Short-term management	Long-term management
Hematocytopenias, including thrombocytopenia and hemolytic anemia (leukopenia usually requires no therapy)	None required if minor **OR** prednisone 30–60 mg/day as required to normalize count	Taper rapidly to 15 mg/day of prednisone, then by 1.0–2.5 mg every 1–2 weeks to none **OR** taper prednisone to every other day (30–120 mg) if necessary and successful	Often none required **OR** every-other-day prednisone in whatever dose required **OR** azathioprine 100–150 mg/day sometimes used
Active nephritis (therapy influenced by urine sediment, renal fuction, renal biopsy, and serologic abnormalities)	Prednisone 30–60 mg/day as required to normalize urine and stabilize renal function **OR** prednisone plus monthly bolus IV cyclophosphamide 500–1000 mg/M² (especially if no response to prednisone after 2–4 weeks)	Taper prednisone to every other day (60–120 mg); withdraw cyclophosphamide after 3–12 months depending on renal status (may reduce to every 2–3 months before withdrawal)	Continue every-other-day prednisone for 6–12 months after disease becomes inactive; then taper to none **OR** azathioprine 100–150 mg/day sometimes used if prednisone withdrawal difficult
Seizures (exclude other causes!)	None for single isolated seizure **OR** prednisone 60 mg/day **OR** prednisone plus anticonvulsant drug	Taper rapidly to 15 mg/day of prednisone and then by 1.0–2.5 mg every 1–2 weeks to none **OR** taper prednisone to every other day (60–120 mg) if necessary	Usually none required **OR** every-other-day prednisone for a few months **OR** anticonvulsant drug if felt to be indicated
"Psychosis" or dementia (exclude steroid psychosis)	Prednisone 30–60 mg/day as necessary **OR** prednisone plus antipsychotic drugs as needed	Taper rapidly to 15 mg/day of prednisone and then by 1.0–2.5 mg every 1–2 weeks to none **OR** taper prednisone to every other day (60–120 mg) if necessary and successful	Usually none required **OR** every-other-day prednisone for a few months and then withdraw gradually

CNS thrombotic events with cardiolipin antibody	Anticoagulation OR anticoagulation plus prednisone 30–60 mg/day	Taper rapidly to 15 mg/day of prednisone, then by 1.0–2.5 mg every 1–2 weeks to none	Long-term anticoagulation is controversial; antiplatelet drugs are less controversial
Severe CNS disease ("cerebritis") with altered mental status and recurrent seizures	Parenteral methylprednisolone 100–1000 mg/day as necessary OR parenteral methylprednisolone plus bolus IV cyclophosphamide as above	Taper rapidly to 60 mg/day of prednisone; then taper to every other day (60–120 mg). Withdraw cyclophosphamide after 3–6 months	Every-other-day prednisone for several months after normal mental status achieved then withdraw gradually
Cutaneous small-vessel (leukocytoclastic) vasculitis	No therapy essential if only cutaneous OR prednisone 15–30 mg/day as necessary	Taper rapidly to 15 mg/day of prednisone; then by 1.0–2.5 mg every 1–2 weeks to none OR taper prednisone to every other day (15–60 mg) if necessary	Usually none required OR every-other-day prednisone as long as necessary OR azathioprine 50–150 mg/day sometimes used
Systemic necrotizing vasculitis (arteritis)	Prednisone 60–120 mg/day or parenteral equivalent OR prednisone plus bolus IV cyclophosphamide as above OR prednisone plus PO cyclophosphamide 100–150 mg/day	Taper prednisone to every other day (80–160 mg); withdraw intravenous cyclophosphamide after 3–6 months; withdraw PO cyclophosphamide after 6–12 months	Continue every-other-day prednisone for 6–12 months; then gradually withdraw OR azathioprine 100–150 mg/day sometimes used
Myocarditis	Prednisone 60–120 mg/day or parenteral equivalent plus standard heart failure therapy	Taper prednisone to every other day (60–120 mg)	Withdraw every-other-day prednisone gradually after several months of normal myocardial function
Symptomatic pulmonary infiltrates (exclude infection!)	Prednisone 30–60 mg/day as required	Taper prednisone rapidly to 15 mg/day and then by 1.0–2.5 mg every 1–2 weeks to none OR taper prednisone to every other day (30–120 mg) if necessary	Usually none required OR every-other-day prednisone as long as necessary

dosing schedules may be necessary to suppress the symptoms around the clock. In this situation it is generally best to begin with a very low dose such as 5 mg/day of prednisone and gradually increase it until a satisfactory response has been achieved. Since there is seldom any virtue in continuing the drug after the manifestations being treated become quiescent, gradual withdrawal should be initiated soon after a satisfactory response is achieved.

When corticosteroids are used for more serious manifestations, different principles apply. Much larger doses are generally thought to be required, but, even in this case, the lower end of the dosage scale might be prescribed first unless the process is immediately life or organ threatening. With the larger doses, efforts to minimize side effects should take precedent over complete suppression of minor symptoms. Whenever possible, once-a-day dosage schedules should be used initially, and attempts at every-other-day schedules are indicated if prolonged maintenance therapy is likely to be required. It is generally possible to taper large doses more rapidly than small doses. If the manifestation appears to be under control, a daily dose of 60 mg of prednisone can be reduced to 40 mg. Then tapering can proceed by 5–10-mg decrements every one to two weeks until a dose of 15 mg/day is reached. Below 15 mg/day, tapering should be more gradual. A similar program can be used to taper from a daily to an every-other-day schedule. Caution will be necessary to avoid confusing transient symptoms of corticosteroid withdrawal with flares in disease activity.

Cytotoxic-Immunosuppressive Agents

Considerable controversy surrounds the use of cytotoxic-immunosuppressive agents for manifestations of SLE. Probably the least controversial role for these drugs is in the context of active lupus nephritis, especially when corticosteroids have failed to suppress the disease activity. In this case monthly bolus intravenous cyclophosphamide is widely considered to be the approach of choice. Oral or intravenous cyclophosphamide also seems to be indicated for corticosteroid-resistant systemic necrotizing vasculitis, and perhaps for other life-threatening manifestations. In these cases, however, systemic corticosteroids remain the initial therapy of choice; the beneficial effects of the cytotoxic-immunosuppressive agents will require time. Consequently cytotoxic-immunosuppressive agents should not be the sole initial therapy for a manifestation immediately threatening to life or an organ.

Some patients with SLE appear to require prolonged or even indefinite systemic corticosteroid therapy for one or more manifestations. In this case a drug with a "steroid-sparing effect" would be desirable, and cytotoxic-immunosuppressive agents are often used with this goal in mind. Before considering the use of such an agent, however, it would be wise to test the hypothesis that prolonged corticosteroid therapy is really necessary. Although tentative observations suggest that low-dose weekly methotrexate might be useful for this purpose, azathioprine has been the immunosuppressive agent most widely used in this context. Daily doses have varied from 50–175 mg. Side effects and precautions are the same in SLE as in

RA. It should be emphasized, however, that the role of and the value of azathioprine in SLE remain a matter of opinion.

RAYNAUD'S PHENOMENON AND THE SCLERODERMA SYNDROMES

Raynaud's Phenomenon

Raynaud's phenomenon may be primary or it may be secondary to local vascular anomalies, drugs, toxins, cryoproteins, or the connective tissue diseases. Secondary Raynaud's phenomenon tends to be more severe than primary and more often requires therapy. Besides intractable symptoms, complications of Raynaud's phenomenon requiring therapy include persisting digital ischemia, digital ulcers, and recurring or persisting digital infections. A number of vasodilating drugs have been reported to benefit Raynaud's phenomenon, but their use is frequently limited by side effects. Among the more promising agents are topical nitroglycerin, prazosin, and the calcium channel blocking agents, especially the latter.

A number of controlled studies have supported the efficacy of nifedipine (usually 30–90 mg/day) and diltiazem (usually 180–360 mg/day). Not only are these agents usually effective, but they are also better tolerated than most other drugs that have been used for the problem. Nifedipine is usually begun in a dose of 30 mg/day, and the dose is gradually increased until benefits are apparent or to a total daily dose of 90–120 mg. Nifedipine may aggravate the lower esophageal dysfunction often encountered in patients with Raynaud's phenomenon. If it appears to do so, diltiazem may be substituted in equivalent doses. Common side effects of the calcium channel blocking agents are summarized in Table 6-4. It may be necessary to treat Raynaud's phenomenon only during the winter or cooler months. If all symptoms disappear, drug withdrawal may be attempted. If a calcium channel blocking agent alone fails, one experience suggests that the addition of prazosin (3 mg/day) might enhance the response. None of these agents is approved by the FDA for use in Raynaud's phenomenon.

Limited Scleroderma

The true scleroderma syndromes occur in two forms: limited and diffuse. Limited scleroderma is often referred to by the acronym CREST (calcinosis, Raynaud's phenomenon, esophageal dysmotility, sclerodactyly, and telangiectasia). This generally benign syndrome usually requires no drug therapy; however, the Raynaud's phenomenon may be sufficiently symptomatic or complicated to justify treating it as discussed previously. One experience has suggested that the extensive subcutaneous calcinosis occasionally encountered may respond to low-dose warfarin (about 1 mg/day).

Systemic Sclerosis

Diffuse scleroderma or systemic sclerosis is a much more serious, though less common, disease. Unfortunately there is no drug therapy of proven value in its overall management, though some specific

Table 6-4. Side effects of nifedipine and diltiazem

Weakness
Dizziness
Flushing
Edema
Muscle cramps
Heartburn/dyspepsia
Headache
Bradycardia*
Heart block (first degree)*
Hypotension
Drug-induced hepatitis
Bleeding due to antiplatelet effect
Rash
Heart block (second degree)*
Heart failure

*With diltiazem only.

manifestations are amenable to certain specific therapies, and some of these may prove to be lifesaving. They are summarized in Table 6-5. Literally dozens of drugs, including colchicine, isoniazid, chlorambucil, azathioprine, and griseofulvin, have been reported to benefit systemic sclerosis, and then, on more careful scrutiny, have been found to be lacking in value.

Since many of the clinical manifestations of the disease in part at least seem to be related to Raynaud's phenomenon, it seems reasonable to treat it, but no controlled trials have yet demonstrated overall benefits. There is an indication that D-penicillamine in doses of about 750–1000 mg/day may benefit the skin and slow the progression of visceral manifestations, especially pulmonary; however, the side effects of this dose are a major limiting factor, and its routine use must await more convincing proof of its efficacy. No drug therapy has proven value for the lung manifestations, though short courses of high-dose corticosteroids are sometimes tried for rapidly progressive disease. There has never been any evidence that systemic corticosteroids favorably influence overall disease course, and some older reports have associated their use with accelerated hypertension. In general systemic sclerosis is the most untreatable of the connective tissue diseases.

POLYMYOSITIS/DERMATOMYOSITIS

Dermatomyositis is simply polymyositis with cutaneous manifestations, and the two conditions will be considered here as one under the name of polymyositis. In general the various manifestations of the disease (muscle, skin, lungs, and heart primarily) are treated the same, but the major clinical problem is usually the myositis. Among rheumatologists in this country, the therapy is relatively standard, though virtually no controlled study has ever been done to support its efficacy, which has been questioned by some.

Corticosteroids, initially in high doses, are the mainstay of drug therapy. Usually 60 mg/day of prednisone is the initial dose. No response in muscle strength or muscle enzymes in one month might

**Table 6-5. Drug therapy
of specfic manifestations of systemic sclerosis**

Manifestations	Treatment
Raynaud's phenomenon	Calcium channel blocking agents
Arthritis-arthralgias and periarthritis	NSAIDs or low-dose systemic corticosteroids
Myositis	Systemic corticosteroids in whatever dose required to normalize strength and muscle enzymes
Lower esophageal dysfunction and resulting reflux	Usual reflux maneuvers plus antacids or H_2 receptor blockers or sucralfate or metoclopramide, or combination of these
Malabsorption syndrome due to functional blind loop	Appropriate antibotics
Accelerated hypertension/renal failure	Vigorous antihypertensive therapy with angiotensin-converting enzyme inhibitors the agents of choice
Cardiac arrhythmias/heart failure	Usual antiarrhythmic and heart failure therapy
Symptomatic pericarditis	NSAIDs (indomethacin) or systemic corticosteroids in whatever dose required

lead to an increase to 80 mg/day. No satisfactory response after an additional one or two months might lead to the addition of an immunosuppressive agent—most often weekly bolus methotrexate. If a satisfactory response (normal muscle strength) to prednisone alone occurs, gradual tapering is begun, following a withdrawal program similar to that employed with high-dose corticosteroids in SLE. If the tapering is interrupted by disease worsening (decreased muscle strength or rise in muscle enzymes), tapering to every other day in equivalent total doses can be attempted. If this approach is unsuccessful, an immunosuppressive agent might be added to the program in an effort to permit continued prednisone withdrawal. One possible approach to overall disease management is diagrammed in Fig. 6-3.

With or without continued immunosuppressive therapy, the majority of surviving patients should be able to discontinue corticosteroids by five years into their disease, though some will require them for the rest of their lives. Some patients will achieve normal muscle strength with continued elevations in muscle enzymes, and controversy exists over whether or not it is necessary to normalize them. A clinical decision is usually made on the basis of drug side effects and doses required to achieve this goal. Other patients will appear to respond satisfactorily to therapy, and then redevelop muscle weakness with normal muscle enzymes; this is usually an indication of superimposed corticosteroid myopathy and indicates steroid withdrawal. If uncertainty exists, a repeat muscle biopsy is frequently helpful.

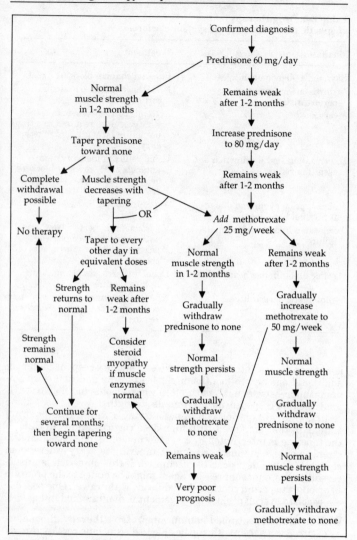

Fig. 6-3. Approach to the drug therapy of polymyositis.

Although a small controlled study has documented delayed and marginal benefits from the addition of azathioprine to a corticosteroid program in polymyositis, most American rheumatologists probably consider methotrexate to be the immunosuppressive agent of choice when corticosteroids fail or cannot be withdrawn. No generally accepted dosage schedule exists, but the drug has usually been given weekly and parenterally. Doses larger than those used in RA are probably required, and 25 mg/week would be a reasonable initial trial dose. If that dose failed, it could be gradually increased to 50 mg/week. Once a response became apparent, corticosteroid withdrawal could be completed before methotrexate withdrawal was attempted. Methotrexate precautions and side effects are the same as in RA, though the larger doses used in polymyositis could be expected to enhance toxicity.

PRIMARY SJÖGREN'S SYNDROME

The prevalence and varied clinical expressions of primary Sjögren's syndrome are just beginning to be appreciated. It appears to be a rather common disorder with a variety of extraglandular manifestations, varying from trivial to serious and life threatening. Moisturizers and lubricants, especially ocular, constitute the most basic therapy and are often the only treatment necessary. Arthralgias and nondestructive arthritis are common and usually respond to NSAIDs, but low-dose corticosteroids are sometimes necessary when NSAIDs are contraindicated. Small-vessel or leukocytoclastic vasculitis is a relatively common manifestation and may require therapy with prednisone in modest doses; usually 15–30 mg/day will suffice and can be tapered rapidly once new cutaneous lesions stop appearing.

More serious manifestations include a variety of CNS syndromes, especially one that resembles multiple sclerosis. This condition has been reported to respond to high-dose prednisone, and a trial of about 60 mg/day is indicated. If a response is apparent, tapering to an every-other-day schedule for a few months of maintenance therapy might be attempted. Systemic necrotizing vasculitis and especially the pseudolymphoma syndrome (extraglandular lymphoproliferation) have been treated with oral cyclophosphamide in doses of 75–100 mg/day with reported successes. Because of the tendency of pseudolymphoma to develop into a lymphoreticular neoplasm, oncologic consultation should be sought when this diagnosis is made. A number of experimental therapies are under investigation, but no definitive one has emerged so far. At this time the most conservative treatment possible is probably the best.

MIXED CONNECTIVE TISSUE DISEASE

Mixed connective tissue disease is an overlapping connective tissue disease syndrome that most often resembles a benign form of SLE. Its therapy is directed at individual manifestations that appear to be active at the time. Maintenance therapy of inactive disease is seldom indicated. Common problems often requiring treatment are summarized in Table 6-6. As a general rule, briefer and less intensive therapy will be required for an expression of mixed connective tissue than would be necessary for the same manifestation of one of the other connective tissue diseases. For example, the myositis associated with this syndrome will usually require lower doses of prednisone for a shorter period of time than would the muscle disease of primary polymyositis. Since the arthritis encountered in mixed connective tissue disease is occasionally destructive, indefinite courses of slow-acting agents will sometimes be indicated, but few other situations require indefinite therapy of any type.

Table 6-6. Drug therapy of common manifestations of mixed connective tissue disease

Manifestation	Therapy
Nonspecific systemic symptoms and low-grade fever	None may be required or short courses of prednisone 5–10 mg/day
Raynaud's phenomenon*	Nifedipine or diltiazem
Nondestructive arthritis	NSAIDs or low-dose prednisone if NSAIDs contraindicated
Destructive arthritis*	Slow-acting agent as in RA
Myositis	Prednisone 30–60 mg/day; taper rapidly once controlled
Pulmonary fibrosis	None of proven value; 1-month trial of prednisone 60 mg/day may be justified if rapidly progressive
Pleuritis/pericarditis	Indomethacin 100–150 mg/day; prednisone 15–30 mg/day if indomethacin contraindicated; taper prednisone rapidly once symptoms controlled
Thrombocytopenia or hemolytic anemia	Prednisone 15–60 mg/day as required; taper prednisone rapidly once blood count normalized

*Indefinite therapy may be required.

Degenerative Joint Diseases

The drug therapy of the degenerative joint diseases (DJDs) is generally unsatisfactory and widely overemphasized by both patients and physicians. Nonpharmacologic approaches such as weight loss, exercise, and various physical therapies are often more beneficial than drugs; however, the pain and disability accompanying DJD may result from more than just mechanical derangements. A secondary synovitis is relatively frequent and may make a significant contribution to the discomfort. The site of the symptoms or the particular joint(s) affected can also be important; hip disease, for example, responds better to drug therapy than does disease of the axial skeleton. The age and general physical condition of the patient are essential considerations, since the elderly and those with certain medical diseases often have contraindications to the use of NSAIDs. Finally there is evidence from animal models of DJD and a few human subjects that certain NSAIDs may actually accelerate cartilage degeneration. Each of these factors must be weighed against the other in designing a rational drug program for patients with DJD.

Asymptomatic DJD requires no medical treatment, though a physical therapy program is sometimes indicated. For those with symptoms, the options include simple analgesics, NSAIDs, and local depot corticosteroids. Systemic corticosteroid therapy is never indicated. The regular use of acetaminophen is probably the safest approach available and may be as satisfactory as any in a surprisingly large number of patients. Narcotic analgesics should be permitted only in low doses and infrequently. Although not very effective, propoxyphene analogs may be the least habit-forming and least toxic of these. NSAIDs may or may not be helpful but are usually tried if no contraindications are present. Almost all NSAIDs marketed in this country have been FDA approved for use in DJD, but only a few trials have compared them to simple analgesics. In most situations lower analgesic doses should be prescribed before resorting to full anti-inflammatory doses, and one of the safer preparations, such as the nonacetylated salicylates, should be tried first. DJD symptoms often wax and wane independent of therapy, and a NSAID prescription need not be indefinite. Intra-articular corticosteroids are controversial in this context; one controlled study failed to demonstrate any benefits of a depot corticosteroid over a local anesthetic. Usually responses are short-lived, and repeated injections risk further damage to articular cartilage and to the joint-supporting structures.

Patients with DJD typically present with a limited number of symptomatic joints—often conforming to distinctive syndromes. These syndromes and the general approaches to their therapy are summarized in Table 6-7. Indomethacin and the hip deserve a special comment; there is some scientific evidence and a large experience to suggest that hip joint DJD often responds better to indomethacin than to other NSAIDs, and the response is sometimes dramatic; therefore, unlike the situation in other DJD syndromes, severe hip pain may justify the risks involved in using this agent, though it should not be the NSAID of first choice and maximum doses should not be used initially. The response of the hip to indomethacin may reflect, in part, the relatively prominent secondary synovitis that occurs at that site. One observation has associated indomethacin use with accelerated cartilage degeneration, however.

Spondyloarthropathies

The two recurring themes in the drug therapy of the spondyloarthropathies are as follows: Indomethacin tends to be the superior NSAID and systemic corticosteroids are often surprisingly ineffective. A number of observations have suggested that phenylbutazone is also more likely to be effective than the other NSAIDs except indomethacin, but it is widely regarded as too toxic for routine and regular use, though short courses may occasionally be permissible. A large experience suggests that salicylates are most often ineffective. Intra-articular corticosteroids are considered by some to be more beneficial in the spondyloarthropathies than in other inflammatory joint diseases, but this apparent benefit may simply reflect the transient nature of the synovitis typical of these disorders; that is, the inflammation may remit on its own before the effects of the injection wear off.

Table 6-7. Overall management of common degenerative joint disease syndromes

Syndrome (site)	Nonpharmacologic therapy (in sequence)	Drug therapy (in sequence)
Heberden's and Bouchard's nodes (hand distal and proximal interphalangeal joints)	Reassurance Physical therapy Surgery seldom indicated	Usually none necessary Simple analgesics Analgesic doses of NSAIDs
Thumb carpometacarpal joint	Splints Physical therapy Surgery (fusion or arthroplasty)	Simple analgesics Analgesic doses of NSAIDs Anti-inflammatory doses of NSAIDs if signs of inflammation Intra-articular corticosteroids sometimes helpful
Inflammatory or erosive osteoarthritis (Heberden's and Bouchard's nodes preceded by synovitis)	Physical therapy Surgery for more severe deformities (usually fusions)	Anti-inflammatory doses of NSAIDs when inflammation present Intra-articular corticosteroids sometimes helpful
Cervical, especially with foraminal nerve root encroachment	Physical therapy, especially traction Surgery (fusion) sometimes necessary	Simple analgesics NSAIDs seldom helpful but may be tried in analgesic doses
Lumbar, especially with spinal stenosis	Physical therapy/exercise Pain clinic/nerve blocks Surgery (decompression/fusion)	Simple analgesics NSAIDs seldom helpful but might be tried in analgesic doses
Hip	Physical therapy/exercises Surgery (arthroplasty)	NSAIDs often helpful, especially indomethacin (see text)
Knee	Weight loss if indicated Physical therapy, especially exercise Support if unstable Surgery (usually arthroplasty)	Simple analgesics Analgesic doses of NSAIDs Intra-articular corticosteroids controversial

PSORIATIC ARTHRITIS

The drug therapy of psoriatic arthritis is, in many ways, similar to the drug therapy of RA. One approach is diagrammed in Fig. 6-4. Several differences between psoriatic arthritis and RA must be considered in designing a drug program, however. These include the generally more benign course, the more episodic nature of the active synovitis, and the typically more limited distribution of the active disease in patients with psoriatic arthritis. Furthermore, in many patients the skin involvement requires as much attention as the joint involvement. Few controlled studies exist of any drug in psoriatic arthritis, and few drugs are specifically FDA approved for use in that context. Consequently the drug therapy of this disease is generally less aggressive and considerably more empiric than the drug therapy of RA.

Once the disease fails to respond adequately to indomethacin and intra-articular corticosteroids, several options are available; however, these will be required in the minority of patients. Enough experience with parenteral gold has been had to suggest that it may be as effective in psoriatic arthritis as in RA, and no evidence shows that it exacerbates the skin disease; however, it does not benefit the skin and there is always uncertainty concerning the duration of therapy in patients responding to it. It may not be necessary to continue it indefinitely, but one is hesitant to stop it and then have to begin all over again a year or two later. Otherwise parenteral gold is used in psoriatic arthritis just as it is used in RA.

In many ways methotrexate is a more appealing drug since it may benefit both the joints and the skin, and its rapid onset of action makes limited courses of therapy more practical. Methotrexate is used in psoriatic arthritis just as it is used in RA, and the same precautions apply **except** that cirrhosis is probably a significantly greater threat in psoriasis than in RA. Pretreatment and more frequent post-treatment liver biopsies have been recommended.

Other long-term therapeutic options must be considered more experimental. One study has demonstrated a response to low-dose daily colchicine. Several reports have suggested benefits from the retinoid etretinate (Tegison), and the drug is FDA approved for use in severe psoriasis; however, it has a number of very common side effects, including alopecia, hyperostosis, stomatitis, dermatitis, bone and joint pain, fever, gastrointestinal symptoms, and visual changes. Doses have varied from 0.5–1.5 mg/kg/day. Other reports also raise a question of whether improved skin disease may lead to improved joint disease; treatment of psoriasis with the photosensitizing agent methoxsalen and long-wave ultraviolet-A light (PUVA) may benefit the joints as well as the skin. Anecdotal reports have also suggested beneficial responses to D-penicillamine, oral zinc sulfate, cimetidine, and cyclosporin.

ANKYLOSING SPONDYLITIS

There is evidence that adequate sustained NSAID therapy of active ankylosing spondylitis improves function and delays axial fusion, perhaps because comfortable patients are more likely to remain physically active. In any event the basic therapy of the disease is a

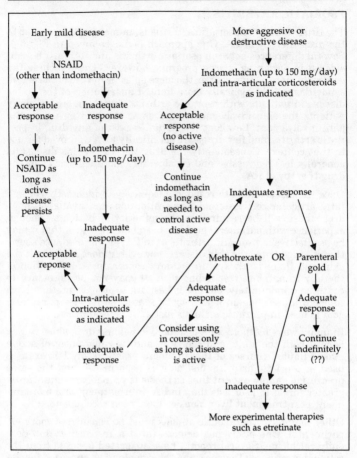

Fig. 6-4. Drug therapy of psoriatic arthritis.

satisfactory NSAID program in conjunction with intensive physical therapy. For decades phenylbutazone was considered to be the NSAID of choice, but indomethacin is now regarded as the preferable drug. If indomethacin cannot be tolerated or is ineffective, short courses of phenylbutazone may be permissible, but it is too toxic for long-term use. Other NSAID alternatives are a matter of opinion, but salicylates are most often ineffective.

Of numerous other agents tried in patients with ankylosing spondylitis, only sulfasalazine seems to offer promise. At least three double-blind controlled studies have suggested a beneficial response over several weeks or months to doses of 2–3 gm/day. Dosing schedules and responses appear to be similar to those in RA, but improvement in patients with ankylosing spondylitis is more difficult to measure. It is yet to be shown that sulfasalazine can significantly delay axial fusion or otherwise alter the overall course of the disease; however, it is generally well tolerated and probably worth trying in patients with obviously progressive disease despite adequate NSAID therapy, and it may be the only reasonable option in patients who cannot tolerate effective NSAIDs.

REITER'S SYNDROME

Included here are all predominantly peripheral spondyloarthropathies not associated with psoriasis. The episodic nature and frequently benign course of many of these syndromes should be considered in designing a drug program. Again indomethacin is probably the most effective NSAID and salicylates probably the least effective; the choice of NSAID is otherwise a matter of opinion. Intraarticular and other intralesional depot corticosteroid injections often appear to result in lasting benefits. In most patients the combination of a satisfactory NSAID program and occasional intralesional injections will be the only drug therapy required.

In the peripheral spondyloarthropathies, second-line agents, when they appear to be required, are often relatively ineffective and there is little scientific basis for their use. One controlled study has suggested delayed benefits from azathioprine, given as it is in RA. Methotrexate has been widely used, but no controlled studies support its efficacy and numerous anecdotes suggest frequent failures. If either of these agents is used, courses rather than indefinite therapy should be planned. The acquired immunodeficiency syndrome has a fairly strong association with Reiter's syndrome, and efforts to exclude the former are indicated before prescribing either azathioprine or methotrexate for the latter.

The role of antibiotic therapy in the peripheral spondyloarthropathies remains controversial, but no controlled studies suggest any benefits in the absence of serologic evidence of Lyme disease, which also may be associated with Reiter's syndrome.

Crystal-Induced Rheumatic Disease

Only acute attacks of articular gout and psuedogout will be considered here, and they can be considered together since the drug therapy of the two conditions is identical. The long-term drug management of the hyperuricemia of gout is discussed in detail elsewhere (see Antihyperuricemic Therapy in Chapter 5). The major factors determining a satisfactory response to the therapy of acute gout/pseudogout are the correct diagnosis and the duration of the attack at the time treatment is initiated. Only the correct diagnoses are likely to respond dramatically to the therapy aimed at them, and they usually depend on crystal identification. Attacks that have persisted for longer than about a week at the time of treatment and the stage of chronic smoldering synovitis achieved by some of these patients before treatment is sought cannot be expected to respond rapidly or dramatically to therapy. In these situations long-term anti-inflammatory drug treatment often will be required.

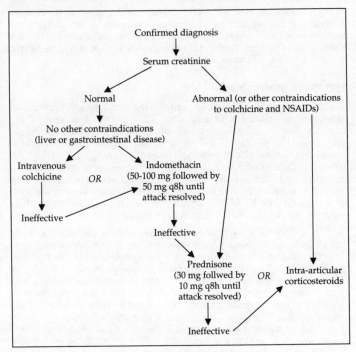

Fig. 6-5. Treatment of acute gout/pseudogout.

Approaches to the treatment of acute gout/pseudogout are summarized in Fig. 6-5. Problems associated with the use of intravenous colchicine have been discussed elsewhere. Although few comparative studies exist, considerable experience suggests that indomethacin is the most effective NSAID (perhaps other than phenylbutazone, which is more toxic). Larger initial doses, such as 100 mg, are likely to be more rapidly effective than smaller doses. Although current textbooks continue to discourage the use of systemic corticosteroids in acute gout/pseudogout, few other options are available when contraindications exist to the use of colchicine and NSAIDs, and recent reports support the efficacy of both prednisone and adrenocorticotropic hormone. Prednisone doses recommended in Fig. 6-5 are estimates based on limited published and personal experience. When intra-articular corticosteroids are the sole therapy of acute gout/pseudogout, attacks may develop in untreated joints. Whichever systemic therapy is employed, it should be withdrawn rapidly after the inflammation has subsided; it can be restarted easily if there is evidence for recurrence. Treatment is seldom necessary for more than 48 hours after an attack has resolved.

Vasculitis Syndromes

Drug therapy of the various vasculitis syndromes is largely empiric since few controlled studies exist. Based on published experiences, two approaches will generally be recommended: systemic corticosteroids or cyclophosphamide, or both, either orally or intravenously. No evidence shows that systemic corticosteroids favorably affect ultimate outcome in patients with these diseases, though they can clearly suppress clinical manifestations, and there is compelling evidence only in the case of Wegener's granulomatosis that cyclophosphamide alters the disease course for the better. For purposes of this discussion, four syndromes will be considered: polyarteritis nodosa, Wegener's granulomatosis, giant-cell arteritis, and the hypersensitivity (leukocytoclastic) vasculitides.

POLYARTERITIS NODOSA

The Churg-Strauss syndrome (or allergic granulomatosis) will also be considered under this category since the therapy is the same as for polyarteritis. A confirmed diagnosis is essential; treatment of presumed unproven polyarteritis is a dangerous trap. High-dose systemic corticosteroids (prednisone 60–100 mg/day) are universally recommended, at least as initial therapy, even though there is evidence that they do not favorably affect survival. A widespread opinion is that cyclophosphamide does favorably affect survival and may even result in a remission though a recent study tended to refute that claim. Consequently it can be recommended for patients who have had life- or organ-threatening manifestations and for patients incompletely responsive to corticosteroids. The usual dose is 1–2 mg/kg/day orally. If a remission is achieved, the prednisone can be tapered to every other day or none (which may unmask cyclophosphamide side effects), and the cyclophosphamide continued for several months to a year. Monthly intravenous bolus cyclophosphamide therapy may have a role, but more experience is required in order to recommend it.

WEGENER'S GRANULOMATOSIS

Although there may be some room for debate, it is relatively clear that cyclophosphamide is not only lifesaving but also remission inducing in patients with Wegener's granulomatosis. Again a definite diagnosis is essential, and an early diagnosis is important, since therapeutic responses are better in patients who have not yet developed renal insufficiency. Initially symptoms should be suppressed with high-dose corticosteroids, which can be tapered to every other day or to none as the disease becomes clinically inactive. There is near-universal agreement that oral cyclophosphamide in a dose of 1–2 mg/kg/day should be started at the time of diagnosis and continued for about a year after remission is clinically apparent. If cyclophosphamide cannot be tolerated, azathioprine in a dose of 2–3 mg/kg/day can be substituted for maintenance after remission is induced. With this program an apparent cure can be expected in most patients treated prior to the onset of renal involvement.

A few reports have suggested apparent remissions in Wegener's granulomatosis induced by trimethoprim-sulfamethoxazole (Bactrim), but there will have to be much more convincing evidence that this agent is effective before it can be recommended as the sole therapy of this highly lethal disease. In any event the effects of the agent appear to be suppressive rather than curative.

GIANT-CELL ARTERITIS AND POLYMYALGIA RHEUMATICA

In this country, giant-cell arteritis is usually seen in the elderly in the form of temporal arteritis. It is a self-limiting illness with an average duration of about four years, and its mortality appears to be negligible; however, active disease carries the significant risk of permanent visual loss and stroke. Consequently, therapy is primarily directed at preventing these complications. The only therapy of obvious value is high-dose corticosteroids (prednisone 60 mg/day), and even this does not shorten the course of the disease, though it is thought to prevent most of the serious complications. High-dose corticosteroids should be used for several weeks to adequately suppress disease activity before tapering is begun. Every-other-day schedules appear to be ineffective. Symptoms, physical findings, and acute-phase reactants can be used to follow the activity of the arteritis as the prednisone is slowly tapered. Many patients will require significant doses for two years or longer, and side effects often become a major clinical problem.

Although the rheumatic pain syndrome of polymyalgia rheumatica is associated with giant-cell arteritis, most patients with the former do not have the latter. Once a diagnosis of polymyalgia rheumatica is made, care must be taken to exclude giant-cell arteritis; if there is no evidence for it, the pain syndrome can be treated symptomatically. Some patients will respond to NSAIDs, but most will probably require low-dose corticosteroids (prednisone 15 mg/day), which are typically dramatically effective. Once the symptoms are controlled, gradual tapering can be begun, but a number of patients will require therapy for two years or longer; like giant-cell arteritis, the course of polymyalgia rheumatica is self-limiting.

HYPERSENSITIVITY VASCULITIS

Synonyms for hypersensitivity vasculitis include allergic vasculitis, leukocytoclastic vasculitis, venulitis, and small-vessel vasculitis. The major target structure is the postcapillary venule, circulating immune complexes most often play a role, the skin is usually affected, and serious extracutaneous manifestations most often occur in the kidney. Numerous associations and causes, including the connective tissue diseases, exist. Consequently it is sometimes difficult to distinguish the manifestations of the vasculitis from the manifestations of the underlying disease. Treatment is highly variable depending on the underlying cause. Therapy of vasculitis in the connective tissue diseases has been addressed in an earlier section of this chapter. Drugs or other antigens that may be precipitating the reaction should be withdrawn or removed from the patient's environment. Mild cases, whatever the cause, may require no therapy or they may respond to brief courses of low-dose corticosteroids. Severe cases, usually with renal involvement, whatever the cause, are usually treated as polyarteritis nodosa would be.

A few specific situations require comment. The prodrome of hepatitis B and some drug reactions present as an acute serum sickness–like reaction with fever, urticaria (vasculitis), and arthritis. These are self-limiting and require only symptomatic therapy, though sometimes short courses of systemic corticosteroids are justified. Henoch-Schönlein purpura is the most common vasculitis of this type seen in children. It is typically benign and self-limiting, requiring only symptomatic therapy; however, short courses of systemic corticosteroids are occasionally indicated, and the disease may be more severe and persisting in adults requiring long-term corticosteroids. The syndrome of essential (idiopathic) mixed cryoglobulinemia tends to be much more serious with severe renal involvement being prominent. When this syndrome appears to be aggressive, it is usually treated like polyarteritis nodosa with corticosteroids and cyclophosphamide.

Juvenile Chronic Arthritis of Unknown Etiology

Juvenile rheumatoid arthritis (JRA) is probably a collection of overlapping syndromes that vary widely in their manifestations and prognosis. For purposes of this discussion, they will be divided into three major patterns: systemic onset, pauciarticular onset, and polyarticular onset. Generally the systemic onset disease, with fever, rash, often destructive polyarthritis, and other extra-articular features, is the most serious of the syndromes and the one that will require the most aggressive therapy. On the other hand, the pauciarticular disease is often benign and self-limiting, typically remitting without serious joint damage during the teenage years; it usually requires only NSAID therapy. The polyarticular-onset pattern often behaves much like adult RA, and it is usually treated like its presumed adult counterpart.

SYSTEMIC ONSET

Systemic-onset JRA, often called Still's disease, may be associated with serious extra-articular manifestations including myocarditis; consequently, therapy is directed at both the systemic disease and the joint disease. An adult counterpart ("adult Still's disease") is fairly common and is treated in much the same way as the juvenile form. Doses of salicylates adequate to produce a therapeutic level (about 75–100 mg/kg/day) are the initial treatment. If salicylates are ineffective or poorly tolerated, naproxen (about 15 mg/kg/day) or tolmetin (about 25 mg/kg/day) have been FDA approved for use in children and might be tried. Serious systemic or extra-articular manifestations, especially when NSAIDs have proven ineffective, are treated with high-dose corticosteroids (prednisone 30–60 mg/day as required). Once the manifestation being treated has been controlled, the prednisone can be tapered over a few months to none or to an every-other-day program. Although the systemic disease often remits in a few months, the joint disease may continue to be progressive and it is destructive in about half of the cases. Aggressive joint disease is an indication for parenteral gold therapy, which probably should be continued indefinitely. If parenteral gold fails, hydroxychloroquine (initially 5–7 mg/kg/day), D-penicillamine (3–10 mg/kg/day in progressive increments), or methotrexate (0.1–0.6 mg/kg/week) might be tried, but the experience with each of these in systemic-onset disease is very limited.

Drug therapy is only one aspect of the treatment of this potentially devastating illness. Hospitalization during the acute phases is often required; intensive occupational and physical therapy is almost always indicated. The best outcome is probably achieved by a multidisciplinary approach during the time the systemic disease is active.

PAUCIARTICULAR ONSET

In younger girls (with antinuclear antibodies), pauciarticular-onset JRA is especially associated with chronic uveitis, which may be a more important consideration than the joint disease. The arthritis of these forms of JRA tends to be nondestructive and is usually treated only with NSAIDs during the time the joint disease is active. Salicylates, naproxen, or tolmetin can be used. If NSAIDs are ineffective or poorly tolerated, judicious use of intra-articular corticosteroids is indicated. Adjunctive physical and occupational therapy may be helpful. More aggressive therapy with systemic corticosteroids or slow-acting agents will rarely be necessary, and very few experiences have been had with slow-acting agents in these syndromes in any event.

POLYARTICULAR ONSET

This pattern of JRA resembles adult RA and its drug therapy is very similar to that of the adult counterpart. Initial treatment consists of NSAIDs, which may be the only therapy required by some patients. Failure to respond to NSAIDs, aggressive joint disease, or systemic symptoms may indicate the need for courses of low-dose corticosteroids (prednisone 15 mg/day or less). Aggressive joint disease will usually require therapy with slow-acting agents. The largest experience is with parenteral gold, but hydroxychloroquine and D-penicillamine may be reasonable alternatives or may be used if parenteral gold fails or cannot be tolerated. A large international study has suggested that auranofin is not beneficial in this syndrome. Small experiences with weekly methotrexate are beginning to appear, and there is a suggestion that relatively larger doses than used in adults may be required for children. A multidisciplinary therapeutic approach, especially involving occupational and physical therapists, can usually be recommended.

Nonarticular or Regional Rheumatic Syndromes

Together the regional rheumatic pain syndromes represent the most common musculoskeletal disorders encountered by primary care physicians. Many of them are undiagnosable and most are transient; consequently their therapy is usually symptomatic. Local myofascial pain syndromes respond poorly to drug therapy but usually resolve on their own in days, weeks, or months. A particularly bothersome regional pain syndrome is a frozen shoulder or adhesive capsulitis that typically defies all efforts at drug and physical therapy. Enthesopathies (inflammation at the site of a connective tissue insertion into bone), tendinitis, and bursitis may be more treatable; these disorders, and two other common regional problems—low back pain and fibromyalgia—will be considered in more detail next.

TENDINITIS, BURSITIS, AND ENTHESOPATHIES

The most common sites for these syndromes are listed in Table 6-8. The onset is typically acute and the diagnosis is usually based on the physical examination. The three therapeutic choices are intralesional depot corticosteroids, NSAIDs, or simple analgesics and physical therapy until the episode resolves on its own. Few scientific studies have addressed these choices, and they remain a matter of opinion. It can be argued that a single depot corticosteroid injection is safer than several days of a NSAID, but largely unfounded concerns over the possibility of tendon damage or rupture continue to be heard. It is probably wise not to inject corticosteroids around the achilles tendon, but a single injection at the other sites appears to be safe. Injections are made around, not into, the tendon. Indomethacin has probably been the most widely used NSAID for these problems, but its superiority in this context has not been proven.

LOW BACK PAIN

Lumbar region or low back pain may be the most common, most undiagnosable, and most untreatable regional musculoskeletal syndrome. The common syndrome is rapid in onset and lacks neurologic or other specific historical and physical features. It usually resolves on its own within a few weeks, but tends to recur. Treatment is nonspecific and symptomatic; no evidence exists that any medical intervention shortens the course of an episode, but exercises and other physical therapy maneuvers may help prevent recurrences. A number of agents, including placebo, seem to offer transient symptomatic relief. Simple analgesics and analgesic doses of NSAIDs are often used for this purpose, but full anti-inflammatory NSAID doses are not indicated. Nonspecific low back pain probably represents the most common reason for prescribing a "muscle relaxant" agent. These drugs may provide some symptomatic relief, but they do not affect the duration of the episode. Their mechanism of action is unknown and their pharmacologic actions are debated; however, these drugs appear to be safe and non-habit-forming. Those commonly used in this country are summarized in Table 6-9. Dantrolene

Table 6-8. Common sites for tendinitis, bursitis, and enthesopathy

Tendinitis
  Rotator cuff (superior shoulder)
  Tendon of long head of biceps (adjacent to shoulder joint)
  Thumb abductor or extensor tendons (near the wrist)
  Achilles tendon (proximal to heel)
Bursitis
  Olecranon (over the elbow)
  Trochanteric (over the trochanter)
  Ischial (over ischial tuberosity)
  Anserine (medial knee)
  Prepatellar (anterior to patella)
Enthesopathy
  Medial epicondyle (of elbow)
  Lateral epicondyle (of elbow)
  Achilles insertion into calcaneum
  Plantal fascia insertion into calcaneum (bottom heel)

Table 6-9. Agents marketed as skeletal muscle relaxants

Generic name	Trade name(s)/size	Dose schedule
Carisoprodol	Soma, 350-mg tablets. Also available generically and in combination with various analgesics.	350 mg tid and at bedtime
Chlorzoxazone	Paraflex, 250-mg tablets. Parafon Forte, 500-mg tablets. Also available generically and in combination with various analgesics.	250–750 mg tid or qid
Cyclobenzaprine	Flexeril, 10-mg tablets. Also available generically.	10 mg tid or qid
Metaxalone	Skelaxin, 400-mg tablets.	800 mg tid or qid
Methocarbamol	Robaxin, 500-mg and 750-mg tablets. Robaxin Injectable, 100 mg/ml. Also available generically and in combination with various analgesics.	Initially 1500 mg qid; maintenance with 500–750 mg tid or qid
		1000 mg IM or IV; may repeat q8hr for 2–3 days

and baclofen (indicated only for spasticity) and those agents used as adjuncts to general anesthesia are not listed. At least one controlled study supports the superiority of cyclobenzaprine in the context of low back pain.

FIBROMYALGIA

Fibromyalgia is the very common chronic generalized musculoskeletal pain syndrome accompanied by tender points at predictable

Table 6-10. Therapeutic options in managing patients with fibromyalgia ("fibrositis")

Education and reassurance
Cardiovascular fitness training program*
Amitriptyline: 25–50 mg at night*
Cyclobenzoprine: 10 mg at night and 1–3 times during the day if needed*
Physical therapies (heat, massage, ultrasound, biofeedback, phonopheresis)
Analgesic doses of NSAIDs or regular acetaminophen for pain relief
Tender point injections if helpful
Patient support groups
Professional psychological help if indicated
Pain clinic referral

*Of proven benefit.

sites that has most often been called "fibrositis." Its therapy is now being actively investigated. Controlled studies, so far, fail to demonstrate any benefits from full anti-inflammatory doses of NSAIDs or from systemic corticosteroid therapy. Available therapeutic options are listed in Table 6-10. Controlled studies have supported the efficacy of two drugs: cyclobenzaprine in various doses (10–40 mg/ day) and amitriptyline usually in doses of 25–50 mg given at night. In these doses, amitriptyline has few serious side effects, but it might be best to begin with 10 mg at night and gradually build up to a satisfactory dose. Other tricyclic antidepressant agents have not been studied but might be expected to be equally effective. Analgesics are almost always required and analgesic doses of NSAIDs are clearly preferable to narcotic analgesics in this syndrome. Tender point injections with a local anesthetic are safe and seem to benefit some patients.

Nondrug therapies may be more important than drug therapies in managing this difficult problem. A controlled study has clearly demonstrated the benefits of a cardiovascular fitness training program, and exercise of any type should be encouraged. Patient education and reassurance are essential. When available, patient support groups also seem to be helpful.

Miscellaneous Rheumatic Diseases

A few miscellaneous rheumatic disorders are not specifically addressed elsewhere in this section. Most of these are relatively uncommon or rare in this country, and their drug therapy is briefly summarized in Table 6-11. A number of other diseases, most notably the endocrinopathies and the hemoglobinopathies, often have rheumatic or articular expressions; however, their therapy is typically the therapy of the underlying disease, and these problems need not be specifically addressed here.

Table 6-11. Drug therapy of miscellaneous uncommon rheumatic diseases

Disease	Therapy	Comment
Amyloidosis	Colchicine about 1 mg/day with or without melphalan, chlorambucil, or cyclophosphamide	No generally accepted or satisfactory therapy; colchicine may prolong survival and is safe
Behçet's disease	High-dose systemic corticosteroids are the mainstay of therapy of active disease; chlorambucil or azathioprine may prevent attacks of or benefit the uveitis and meningoencephalitis	Few controlled studies and no generally satisfactory therapy. Small series suggest benefits from cyclosporin and other immunomodulating agents. Chlorambucil is the most widely used immunosuppressive drug.
Eosinophilic fasciitis	Courses of prednisone 30–60 mg/day for progressive disease	May remit on its own
Familial Mediterranean fever	Colchicine 0.6 mg bid or tid. Treatment of acute attacks is symptomatic	Colchicine prevents attacks and the complication of amyloidosis
Hypertrophic osteoarthropathy	Symptomatic; NSAIDs are often helpful	Underlying cause should be sought and treated

Inflammatory bowel disease arthropathy	NSAIDs if not contraindicated; intra-articular depot corticosteroids; low-dose systemic corticosteroids sometimes necessary	Often responds to the therapy of the underlying bowel disease
Polychondritis	High-dose systemic corticosteroids are the mainstay of therapy for the acute episodes; NSAIDs might be used for joint and other minor symptoms	Anecdotal reports of responses to dapsone, azathioprine, 6-mercaptopurine, and cyclophosphamide in varying doses
Rheumatic fever	Aspirin in full therapeutic doses is mainstay of therapy. Short courses of high-dose systemic corticosteroids are sometimes used for the carditis. Antibiotic prophylaxis is essential.	Dramatic response to salicylates may be helpful diagnostically. Neither NSAIDs nor corticosteroids alter course of disease.
Sarcoid arthritis with erythema nodosum	NSAIDs, especially indomethacin, or low-dose systemic corticosteroids if NSAIDs fail	Therapy should benefit both skin and joints
Chronic granulomatous sarcoid arthritis	NSAIDs, especially indomethacin; intra-articular depot corticosteroids if NSAIDs fail; low-dose systemic corticosteroids occasionally necessary	Oral colchicine has been reported to be effective. Anecdotal reports suggest methotrexate and antimalarials may be effective.

Bibliography

RHEUMATOID ARTHRITIS

Baker, D. G., Rabinowitz, J. L. Current concepts in the treatment of rheumatoid arthritis. *J. Clin. Pharmacol.* 26:2–21, 1986.

Boers, M., and Ramsden, M. Long-acting drug combinations in rheumatoid arthritis: a formal overview. *J. Rheumatol.* 18:316–324, 1991.

Felson, D. T., Anderson, J. J., and Meenan, R. F. The comparative efficacy and toxicity of second-line drugs in rheumatoid arthritis: results of two metaanalyses. *Arthritis Rheum.* 33:1449–1461, 1990.

Frank, R. G., et al. Antidepressant analgesia in rheumatoid arthritis. *J. Rheumatol.* 15:1632–1638, 1988.

Fries, J. F. Reevaluating the therapeutic approach to rheumatoid arthritis: the "sawtooth" strategy. *J. Rheumatol.* (suppl. 22)17:12–15, 1990.

Harris, E. D., Jr. Management of Rheumatoid Arthritis. In W. N. Kelley et al. (eds.), *Textbook of Rheumatology*. Philadelphia: Saunders, 1989. Pp. 982–992.

Weiss, M. M. Corticosteroids in rheumatoid arthritis. *Semin. Arthritis Rheum.* 19:9–21, 1989.

SYSTEMIC LUPUS ERYTHEMATOSUS

Austin, H. A., III, et al. Therapy of lupus nephritis. Controlled trial of prednisone and cytotoxic drugs. *N. Engl. J. Med.* 314:614–619, 1986.

Felson, D. T., and Anderson, J. Evidence for the superiority of immunosuppressive drugs and prednisone over prednisone alone in lupus nephritis. *N. Engl. J. Med.* 311:1528–1533, 1984.

Lehman, T. J. A., Sherry, D. D., and Wagner-Weiner, L. Intermittent intravenous cyclophosphamide therapy for lupus nephritis. *J. Pediatr.* 114:1055–1066, 1989.

McCune, W. J., et al. Clinical and immunologic effects of monthly administration of intravenous cyclophosphamide in severe systemic lupus erythematosus. *N. Engl. J. Med.* 318:1423–1431, 1988.

Steinberg, A. D. The treatment of lupus nephritis. *Kidney Int.* 30:769–787, 1986.

OTHER CONNECTIVE TISSUE DISEASES

deClerck, L. S., et al. D-penicillamine therapy and interstitial lung disease in scleroderma. *Arthritis Rheum.* 30:643–650, 1987.

Plotz, P. H., Dalakas, M., and Leff, R. L. Current concepts in the idiopathic inflammatory myopathies: polymyositis, dermatomyositis, and related disorders. *Ann. Intern. Med.* 111:143–157, 1989.

Sharp, G. C., and Singsen, B. H. Mixed Connective Tissue Disease. In D. J. McCarty (ed.), *Arthritis and Allied Conditions. A Textbook of Rheumatology* (11th ed.). Philadelphia: Lea & Febiger, 1989. Pp. 1080–1091.

Talal, N. Sjögren's Syndrome and Connective Tissue Diseases Associated with Other Immunologic Disorders. In D. J. McCarty (ed.), *Arthritis and Allied Conditions. A Textbook of Rheumatology* (11th ed.). Philadelphia: Lea & Febiger, 1989. Pp. 1197–1213.

Whaley, K., and Alspaugh, M. A. Sjögren's Syndrome. In W. N. Kelley et al. (eds.), *Textbook of Rheumatology*. Philadelphia: Saunders, 1989. Pp. 999–1019.

White, C. J., Phillips, W. A., and Abrahams, L. A. Objective benefit of nifedipine in the treatment of Raynaud's phenomenon. *Am. J. Med.* 80:623–625, 1986.

Wollheim, F. A., and Akesson, A. Treatment of systemic sclerosis in 1988. *Semin. Arthritis Rheum.* 18:181–188, 1989.

DEGENERATIVE JOINT DISEASE

Bland, J. H. Diagnosis and treatment of osteoarthritis. *Curr. Opinion Rheumatol.* 1:315–324, 1989.

Buchanan, W. W., and Kean, W. F. Implications of antirheumatic drug therapy in elderly patients with osteoarthritis. *J. Rheumatol.* (suppl. 14)14:98–100, 1987.

Friedman, D. M., and Moore, M. E. The efficacy of intraarticular steroids in osteoarthritis: A double-blind study. *J. Rheumatol.* 7:850–856, 1980.

Rashad, S., et al. Effect of nonsteroidal anti-inflammatory drugs on the course of osteoarthritis. *Lancet* 2:519–521, 1989.

SPONDYLOARTHROPATHIES

Calin, A. A placebo controlled, crossover study of azathioprine in Reiter's syndrome. *Ann. Rheum. Dis.* 45:653–655, 1986.

Dougados, M., Boumier, P., and Amor, B. Sulphasalazine in ankylosing spondylitis: a double-blind controlled study in 60 patients. *Br. Med. J.* 293:911–914, 1986.

Lally, E. V., and Ho, G., Jr. A review of methotrexate therapy in Reiter's syndrome. *Semin. Arthritis Rheum.* 15:139–145, 1985.

Nissila, M., et al. Sulfasalazine in the treatment of ankylosing spondylitis. *Arthritis Rheum.* 31:1111–1116, 1988.

Richter, M. B., Kinsella, P., and Corbett, M. Gold in psoriatic arthropathy. *Ann. Rheum. Dis.* 39:279–280, 1980.

Seideman, P., Fjellner, B., and Johannesson, A. Psoriatic arthritis treated with oral colchicine. *J. Rheumatol.* 14:777–779, 1987.

Willkens, R. F., et al. Randomized, double-blind, placebo controlled trial of low-dose pulse methotrexate in psoriatic arthritis. *Arthritis Rheum.* 27:376–381, 1984.

CRYSTAL-INDUCED RHEUMATIC DISEASE

Alvarellos, A., and Spilberg, I. Colchicine prophylaxis in pseudogout. *J. Rheumatol.* 13:804–805, 1986.

Boss, G. R., and Seegmiller, J. E. Hyperuricemia and gout. *N. Engl. J. Med.* 300:1459–1468, 1979.

Groff, G. D., Franck, W. A., and Raddatz, D. A. Systemic steroid therapy for acute gout: A clinical trial and review of the literature. *Semin. Arthritis Rheum.* 19:329–336, 1990.

Simkin, P. A. Management of gout. *Ann. Intern. Med.* 90:812–816, 1979.

VASCULITIS SYNDROMES

DeRemee, R. A., McDonald, T. J., and Weiland, L. H. Wegener's granulomatosis: Observations on treatment with antimicrobial agents. *Mayo Clin. Proc.* 60:27–32, 1985.

Fauci, A. S., et al. Wegener's granulomatosis: Prospective clinical and therapeutic experience with 85 patients for 21 years. *Ann. Intern. Med.* 98:76–85, 1983.

Fauci, A. S., et al. Cyclophosphamide therapy of severe systemic necrotizing vasculitis. *N. Engl. J. Med.* 301:235–238, 1979.

Geltner, D. Therapeutic approaches in mixed cryoglobulinemia. *Springer Semin. Immunopathol.* 10:103–113, 1988.

Guillevin, L., et al. Long term followup after treatment of polyarteritis nodosa and Churg-Strauss angiitis with comparison of steroids, plasma exchange and cyclophosphamide to steroids and plasma exchange. A prospective randomized trial of 71 patients. *J. Rheumatol.* 18:567–574, 1991.

Kyle, V., and Hazleman, B. L. Treatment of polymyalgia rheumatica and giant cell arteritis. I. Steroid regimens in the first two months. II. Relation between steroid dose and steroid associated side effects. *Ann. Rheum. Dis.* 48:658–661, 662–666, 1989.

JUVENILE RHEUMATOID ARTHRITIS

Brewer, E. J., et al. Penicillamine and hydroxychloroquine in the treatment of severe juvenile rheumatoid arthritis. *N. Engl. J. Med.* 314:1269–1276, 1986.

Giannini, E. H., et al. Auranofin in the treatment of juvenile rheumatoid arthritis. *Arthritis Rheum.* 33:466–476, 1990.

Grondin, C., Malleson, P., and Petty, R. E. Slow-acting antirheumatic drugs in chronic arthritis of childhood. *Semin. Arthritis Rheum.* 18:38–47, 1988.

Manners, P. J., and Ansell, B. M. Slow-acting antirheumatic drug use in systemic onset juvenile chronic arthritis. *Pediatrics* 77:99–103, 1986.

Rosenberg, A. M. Advanced drug therapy for juvenile rheumatoid arthritis. *J. Pediatr.* 114:171–178, 1989.

NONARTICULAR OR REGIONAL RHEUMATIC SYNDROMES

Bennett, R. M., et al. A comparison of cyclobenzaprine and placebo in the management of fibrositis. *Arthritis Rheum.* 31:1535–1542, 1988.

Frymoyer, J. W. Back pain and sciatica. *N. Engl. J. Med.* 318:291–300, 1988.

Goldenberg, D. L., Felson, D. T., and Dinerman, H. A randomized, controlled trial of amitriptyline and naproxen in the treatment of patients with fibromyalgia. *Arthritis Rheum.* 29:1371–1377, 1986.

Larsson, L., and Baum, J. The syndromes of bursitis. *Bull. Rheum. Dis.* 36:1–8, 1986.

Petri, M., et al. Randomized, double-blind, placebo-controlled study of the treatment of the painful shoulder. *Arthritis Rheum.* 30:1040–1045, 1987.

White, R. H., Paull, D. M., and Fleming, K. W. Rotator cuff tendinitis: Comparison of subacromial injection of a long acting corticosteroid versus oral indomethacin therapy. *J. Rheumatol.* 13:608–613, 1986.

MISCELLANEOUS RHEUMATIC DISEASES

Benson, M. D. Treatment of al amyloidosis with melphalan, prednisone, and colchicine. *Arthritis Rheum.* 29:683–687, 1986.

Cohen, A. S., Rubinow, A., and Anderson, J. J. Survival of patients with primary (AL) amyloidosis. *Am. J. Med.* 82:1182–1190, 1987.

O'Duffy, J. D., Robertson, D. M., and Goldstein, N. P. Chlorambucil in the treatment of uveitis and meningoencephalitis of Behcet's disease. *Am. J. Med.* 76:75–84, 1984.

Yazici, H., et al. A controlled trial of azathioprine in Behçet's syndrome. *N. Engl. J. Med.* 322:281–285, 1990.

Zemer, D., et al. Colchicine in the prevention and treatment of the amyloidosis of familial Mediterranean fever. *N. Engl. J. Med.* 314:1001–1005, 1986.

Index